SIDE EFFECT:
SKINNY

DENISE AUSTIN

SIDE EFFECT:
SK NNY

DENISE AUSTIN'S **FAT-BLAST** DIET

bird
st.
books

Published in Los Angeles, California, by Bird Street Books, Inc.

ISBN: 978-0-9854627-2-7

Cover Design: Eric D. Wilkinson
Interior Design: Maureen Forys, Happenstance Type-O-Rama

Note to Readers: This book is comprised of the opinions and ideas of its author, who is not a medical or health professional, and is meant solely for informational and entertainment purposes. The author and publisher are not providing medical, health, or any other kind of personal professional services within this book. The ideas and concepts in this book are not intended to diagnose, treat, cure, or prevent any health problem or condition, nor are they meant to substitute for professional medical advice. Furthermore, the reader should always consult his or her medical, health, or other competent professional before utilizing any of the concepts in this book. The author and publisher are not, in any way, responsible for any liability, loss, or risk, personal or otherwise, which is incurred as a consequence, directly or indirectly, of the use and application of any of the contents of this book.

With the most humble of hearts for the blessing of such a wonderful family, I dedicate this book to my sweet husband, Jeff, who always puts our family first; and to the true joys in my life, my daughters, Kelly and Katie.

ACKNOWLEDGEMENTS

When it comes to thanking people, I always think of my mom first and foremost. My mom has always been my real-life hero. Her love and devotion to all of us kids and all her grandchildren remain an inspiration. Her enthusiasm for life and encouragement will live in me forever. I miss my mom every day. To my dad, who taught me many valuable lessons, but he especially ingrained in me a strong work ethic. To my husband, Jeff, my "honey bunny," who still makes me laugh even after being married for 29 years. Being a mom is my favorite thing in life. I am so grateful for my healthy and happy daughters, Kelly and Katie. They have become such amazing, smart and wonderful young adults, and I am so proud of them, and I love them so much. And a forever thanks to all three of my sisters and my brother who have shaped who I am today. I love our close-knit family—that's what life is all about—family and friends.

I want to thank Deb Bruce for all her help with this book—she was so awesome to work with. Also, a big thanks to our dietician, Judy Kaplan, MS, RD, for helping me plan out such healthy meals. I am so thankful to Jay McGraw, Scott Waterbury, and Lisa Clark for making this book happen. They have all be so great and so fun. A very special thanks to Jan Miller and Nena Madonia, my literary agents and dear friends—I love you guys.

I have so many wonderful girlfriends that have helped me in some way with this book and I want to thank you: Susan Shaw, Margaret Bush, Debra Swan, Becky Quinn, Deb Johns, Susie Carlson, Kathy Kernochan, Geri Newburn, Mindy Kole, MaryBeth Dyson, Lisa Wheeler, Debbie Strong, and of course my sisters, Kristine, Anne and Donna. I love you all.

DISCLAIMER

This book is comprised of the opinions and ideas of its author, who is not a medical or health professional. The contents of this book is meant solely for general informational and entertainment purposes on the subjects addressed in the book. The author and publisher are not engaged in the rendering of medical, health, psychological, therapeutic, or any other kind of personal professional services within this book. The ideas and concepts in this book are not intended to diagnose, treat, cure, or prevent any medical, health, mental, or psychological problem or condition, nor are they meant to substitute for professional advice of any kind. Furthermore, the reader should always consult his or her medical, health, or other competent professional before utilizing any of the concepts in this book. The author and publisher specifically disclaim all responsibility for, and are not liable for, any liability, loss, or risk, personal or otherwise, which is incurred as a consequence, directly or indirectly, of the use and application of any of the contents of this book.

CONTENTS

INTRODUCTION

Welcome to *Side Effect: Skinny*. This book represents everything I've learned about losing weight, getting fit, banishing belly fat, and boosting good health. It doesn't matter what your dieting history is, how many past attempts you've made at weight loss, what your current fitness level is, or even your age, you *can* get healthy, sexy, and strong. And I'll be right here by your side, cheering you on every step of the way. I want to get you on the right track to feeling amazing because YOU are worth it!

How many times have you wished you had a flatter tummy, or a smaller butt, or thinner thighs, or tighter underarms? You're not alone. Most women I've spoken to around the globe express the very same frustrations—wanting tried-and-true ways to lose excess fat once and for all, so they can feel and look great in their own body.

I've been promoting health and fitness for more than 25 years, and I'm so passionate about making a difference in the lives of women. I completely understand weight problems, I promise you; I've heard every story and seen it all. And I'm no exception—of course I go through times when it's hard to control everything I eat or make time for exercise, especially when I'm traveling or enjoying big gatherings with family or friends. I know it's not easy. My speaking engagements and TV schedule keep me constantly juggling career and family responsibilities, so I understand what it's like to be a little short on time, but I'm going to show you how to work around that and still get fit!

My enthusiasm for fitness started at a young age. At the age of 12, I discovered my love for gymnastics, and spent my teenage years competing in gymnastic events across the US. I was awarded an athletic scholarship to the University of Arizona, where I continued to compete in college gymnastics and received a Bachelor of Arts degree in physical education, with an emphasis in exercise physiology.

At the University of Arizona, the exercise physiology department staff did all their body fat testing on the college gymnastic team. I was essentially one of their guinea pigs, going underwater hooked up to all sorts of body-fat testing devices and being connected to the oxygen capacity test on the treadmill. This was the first time I had ever heard of body-fat testing, and I was enthralled with this research. I knew then that I wanted to learn all I could about the human body. My last year of college, I did a year-long intensive research program on corporate fitness at California State University at Long Beach.

After graduating from college, I couldn't wait to start my career in the fitness industry. I started teaching aerobics at corporate giants such as Kaiser, Northrop, and TRW. Each day of the work week, I got up before 5 a.m., went to the cafeteria of each company, moved the tables and chairs, and started helping the employees learn how to exercise properly, burn calories, and get back in shape. I loved every minute of it. I thought, "This is what I was meant to do."

I wanted to tell the world what I'd learned about keeping the body fit and healthy. I started teaching more aerobic exercise classes in the Los Angeles area and then went on to host several top TV shows starting on the Jack LaLane Show. I served as the fitness expert on NBC's Today Show and produced my first workout videos, *Rock Aerobics* and *Rock Hard Tummy*. Since then, I've created more than 100 workout videos and DVDs and written 14 books on weight loss, fitness, and health. I have served two terms on the President's Council on Physical Fitness and Sports—all in an effort to help people just like you lose that weight and get super healthy again.

While I have dedicated my life to teaching people all around the world how to get fit, I'm not immune to weight fluctuations, just like other women. After the births of my two beautiful daughters, Kelly and Katie, in the 90s, I had to deal with getting back in shape again. I gained around 35 pounds with each pregnancy, but only lost 10 pounds after each delivery. Wow! That was the big wake-up call that I needed to change the way I was eating and exercising to lose the extra baby fat and get trim and healthy again.

While caring for my kids, and with my TV career and other commitments, I made some easy changes in my daily calorie intake and worked in extra time for interval exercises—a series of low- to high-intensity exercise workouts—while pushing the girls in their strollers twice a day, and doing my own favorite aerobic routines while they napped. I was determined to make my physical fitness a priority, despite my busy schedule.

Then I hit my mid-40s. And like most women at this age, my once-reliable body started betraying me. I could no longer eat the same foods without gaining a pound or two, and inevitably it would go right to my belly or thighs! Even the chocolate chip cookies I made for my family were hard to resist, yet I knew if I didn't say "no," I would end up wearing them on my tummy. Not only did I have to revamp my calorie intake again, but I also had to modify my exercise regimen to stay slim.

I, too, have had to kick-start my metabolism, blast the fat, and take it up a notch. In doing so, I've enjoyed the amazing skinny side effects of losing excess pounds, keeping my tummy and thighs trim, and most importantly, looking and feeling fantastic.

You deserve those kinds of side effects, too. Your success is my ultimate motivation for writing this book. My approach in *Side Effect: Skinny* is sensible, fun, and realistic. I'm not asking you to skip meals, eat weird or boring foods, or work out till you drop. Instead, I want to empower you with knowledge about your own body and show you the importance of taking time for yourself each day. Most importantly, I want you to realize that you are *worth* the time it takes to get healthy.

I believe it's all about your attitude. I don't want you to let your life get blocked by negativity. Instead, it's time to get positive about weight loss. Being positive is a choice, and it becomes a habit over time. You can choose to eat the right foods, think optimistically, embrace physical activity, and love your body. Your mantra will be: I can do it. I will do it. I must do it!

Life is such a gift. My ultimate goal is to help you enjoy life, each and every day. I want you to feel so much better about yourself, to look and feel healthier and happier and more satisfied with your body and life. As you begin this weight-loss program, I encourage you to surround yourself with family and friends who will support you with the *Side Effect: Skinny* program. I believe we all must approach difficult tasks with a positive attitude in order to succeed, and that success will inspire others. Your enthusiasm will become infectious.

I seriously believe that we age because we don't stay fit. But you can go from fat to fit at any age. By integrating exercise into your daily lifestyle, you can stay young, look young, and feel young.

In *Side Effect: Skinny*, you will find the simple tools you need for weight-loss success. I can't wait to hear from you as you drop the pounds, get fit, and most importantly, get healthy again.

CHAPTER 1

WHY *SIDE EFFECT: SKINNY* IS THE DIET PLAN FOR YOU

Getting healthy is the best gift you can give yourself!
—Denise

Most of us will have times in our lives when the extra pounds start to pile on. It seems inevitable, doesn't it? You may go to bed one night and feel in control of your life, and then wake up to unattractive, bulging hips the next day. Or like so many women I talk to, the added pounds may go straight to your tummy, causing the dreaded muffin top. Luckily for you, those are exactly the areas we are going to target. In just a few weeks, you can lose that fat around your hips and belly.

Maybe you gained an extra 15 pounds with your first pregnancy and no matter how hard you try, you can't lose them. Or perhaps you added another 10 pounds when the kids left home or when you transitioned into menopause. I get it. No matter when or why you gained weight, I want you to know that *you are not alone*. I have exciting answers in *Side Effect: Skinny* that will change your weight, your health, and your life... forever.

Recently, I was traveling around the country, and it became quite apparent to me that the obesity crisis in the United States has hit epidemic proportions. Over half of the people I saw or spoke to in 11 different cities were overweight or obese. When I returned home, I talked to a Mayo Clinic doctor about my perception. She confirmed that the obesity rates in the United States have soared, particularly over the past 3 decades, saying more than 65 percent of Americans are overweight and one-third of the United States population is classified as obese. These numbers were a huge wake-up call for me, as they should be for you.

 LOSE BELLY FAT AT MENOPAUSE

After menopause, you begin to store fat in your abdomen rather than in your thighs, butt, and hips, because of a drop in a type of estrogen called estradiol, but you maintain levels of another type of estrogen, called estrone, which is directly correlated to fat storage. Many women also lose muscle mass, which further decreases metabolism. But don't throw your hands up in despair! You don't *have* to gain fat after menopause. My Interval Walking Program can help reverse this weight gain and boost your metabolism permanently.

7 HEALTH PROBLEMS CAUSED BY BEING OVERWEIGHT

"But what if I only need to lose 5 or 10 pounds?" If that's the case, you certainly aren't considered obese. But even if you're in a healthy weight range, you could still carry around dangerous belly fat. Now I'm not talking about a little pooch above your belt that you hide with just the right top. I'm referring to the visceral fat in the abdomen that wraps around and squeezes your internal organs. While subcutaneous fat is noticeable because it supports your skin, visceral fat lies deep within the abdominal muscles. This type of fat is metabolically active (it interacts with the process of metabolism), producing dangerous hormones that can damage your health, leading to a host of serious, even life-threatening problems, including:

▶ High blood pressure, which is elevated pressure in the arteries; a risk factor for stroke and heart disease.

▶ High LDL ("bad") cholesterol. LDL cholesterol is a waxy, fat-like substance in the blood that increases the risk of heart disease and stroke if it's too high. You want your HDL ("good") cholesterol to be high and your LDL cholesterol to be low.

▶ High triglycerides. Triglycerides are a type of blood fat that boost the process of atherosclerosis, or, hardening of the arteries.

▶ Metabolic syndrome, which is a group of conditions, including high blood pressure, high blood glucose, abnormal cholesterol, and excess body fat, that increases the risk of stroke, diabetes, and heart disease.

 APPLE OR PEAR?

Scientists tend to categorize women based on where they carry fat. Women who gain mainly around their mid-sections, but stay thin everywhere else, are referred to as apple-shaped. Women whose fat goes to their lower bodies, namely their butts and thighs, are pear-shaped. Medically speaking, it's more dangerous to be apple-shaped, as this abdominal fat places you at a higher risk for several life-threatening conditions, such as diabetes, heart disease, stroke, high blood pressure, and even some cancers. Of course, these health conditions aren't written in stone. You have the power to change your apple shape by starting the 7-Day Fat-Blast Diet and Workout to lose the extra belly fat and reduce your chance of developing serious health problems.

DO YOU HAVE HIGH BLOOD PRESSURE?

Did you know that 1 out of every 3 adults in the US has high blood pressure (hypertension)? Because high blood pressure has no early warning signs, most people do not know they have it until they see their doctor. High blood pressure can go unnoticed and untreated for years, damaging your kidneys, heart, and other organs—even causing a stroke. Your doctor should check your blood pressure every 2 years. Many pharmacies and blood drives offer blood pressure checks, too, or consider getting a blood pressure monitor for your home. The good news: modest weight loss may bring your blood pressure down to normal.

- ▶ Type 2 diabetes, which is caused by either a lack of insulin or the body's inability to efficiently use the insulin it produces.

  - ■ The more visceral fat you have, the greater your risk of type 2 diabetes.

  - ■ In fact, more than 80 percent of people with type 2 diabetes, the most common type of the disease, are obese or overweight.

- ▶ Sleep apnea, which is the cessation of breathing that may occur during sleep.

- ▶ Cancer—the uncontrolled growth of abnormal cells in the body that can be life threatening. Cancer is the second leading cause of death in women.

Not only are obesity and belly fat major health challenges for most Americans, but, in my opinion, the latest diets and fads have failed to provide lasting results. Maybe you've tried one (or several) of those diets and you lost a few pounds the first few weeks. But then you hit that stubborn weight-loss plateau where the scales simply wouldn't budge anymore. No matter how much you exercised or starved yourself, your weight stayed the same. The reason? Your body became accustomed to the number of calories on the diet and halted any weight-loss efforts. I have heard this repeatedly from so many women, including women I meet in seminars, my girlfriends, and those who visit my website (*www.DeniseAustin.com*).

 ## TEST YOUR BLOOD SUGAR

Diabetes increases your risk of heart disease, kidney disease, vision problems, stroke, and other very serious conditions. Getting your blood sugar checked by your doctor regularly is a good way to prevent these health problems. If you have diabetes, stay on your prescribed medications and follow your doctor's recommendations for diet and exercise. The good news: dropping pounds lowers blood sugar and may help you get off type 2 diabetes medications.

 ## CHOLESTEROL SCREENING

Your doctor will test your *lipid profile*, which includes the levels of all the different types of cholesterol and fats in your bloodstream. Many doctors recommend that their patients have this lipid profile test at age 45 and then every 5 years after that. If you have any risk factors for heart disease, your doctor will want to test your lipid profile at a younger age. Also, if you have a family history of high cholesterol levels, ask your doctor to check your lipid profile. The good news: Losing 5 to 10 percent of your body weight can greatly reduce your cholesterol levels. Remember, LDL ("bad") cholesterol increases your risk of heart disease when it is high; HDL ("good") cholesterol lowers the chance of heart disease when it is high. So, you always want your LDL cholesterol to be low and your HDL cholesterol to be high.

Did your doctor suggest that you lose weight to lower your blood pressure or LDL cholesterol? That has happened to many women I know as they get older, and, sure enough, once they dropped 10 or 15 pounds, their blood pressure and LDL cholesterol level dropped too. Maybe you have read that losing just 15 pounds would reduce chronic joint pain with osteoarthritis, ease lower back pain, or reduce the risk of developing type 2 diabetes or even some types of cancer. It's true.

But why have you gained weight? Stress eating? Nighttime eating? Snacking during PMS? The real reason you gain weight is simple: You eat more calories than you burn (or you burn fewer calories than you eat).

To gain a pound, you must eat 3500 more calories than you burn through exercise and physical activity. To lose a pound—you guessed it—you must burn 3500 calories more than you eat. Yes, I'm talking about basic math—to lose weight, you need to eat less and exercise more. If you're groaning because that sounds too hard, just stick with me. I'm going to show you how to eat fewer of the foods that slow your weight loss and more foods that speed up the efficiency with which your body torches calories, without starving. Hey, I like to eat, and I'm sure you do, too. Starvation diets don't keep the weight off in the long run anyway, so why bother feeling hungry all the time?

 TYPE 2 DIABETES IS AN EPIDEMIC

Type 2 diabetes is a worldwide epidemic today. It is estimated by the World Health Organization (WHO) that 346 million people around the globe have type 2 diabetes. According to the WHO, diabetes is on track to be one of the top 10 leading causes of death globally by 2030. Again, losing weight reduces the risk of type 2 diabetes. If you are a woman with type 2 diabetes, weight loss and exercise can improve your blood glucose levels and reduce the need for diabetes medications.

This diet can help you kick your metabolism into high gear, so you can burn calories even faster and lose the extra weight. The concepts in this book are based on *Calorie Confusion*, which switches up your caloric intake every 2 days to help trick your metabolism, so you can blast the fat.

Metabolism is your body's process for turning calories into energy—and it varies for each woman and even at different life stages. The faster your metabolic rate, the faster your body burns calories, which means they are not going to land on your belly or hips.

Metabolism drops 1 to 2 percent every year after age 20. Sorry, ladies; it's just a fact of life. The problem is that with aging, the amount of muscle also begins to decline and fat starts to account for more of your weight. More fat and less muscle is a perfect recipe for obesity, because it slows down calorie burn, or your basal metabolic rate, resulting in added pounds, including belly fat.

Monthly hormonal changes with premenstrual syndrome (PMS) can lead to weight gain if you give in to your carbohydrate cravings at that time of the month (many women crave foods with high carbs like desserts, fast food, and so on during this time of month). Also, hormonal changes in your 40s and 50s can definitely cause you to gain weight. For instance, gaining weight during perimenopause and menopause could also be the result of a loss of muscle mass and decreased

 ## REDUCE YOUR RISK OF BREAST CANCER

If you're 40 years old or older, you should talk to your doctor about having a mammogram—an x-ray of your breasts. Mammograms detect tumors that might be too small to feel during breast exams. Early detection offers the best chance at successful treatment. Be sure to perform your monthly breast self-exams and talk to your doctor immediately if you notice any changes. The good news: lowering estrogen levels by losing weight reduces your chance of estrogen-sensitive breast cancer by about 50 percent. That's some great motivation to stay on track!

activity level that may accompany aging (but does not have to!). Again, being inactive and having less muscle leads to added pounds. Also giving in to the temptation of comfort foods—brownies, white bread, and junk food—in response to uncomfortable menopausal symptoms such as hot flashes, night sweats, and irritability easily leads to weight gain.

The good news is that exercise increases muscle mass and boosts your body's metabolic rate, both of which are necessary for losing weight. Also, exercise helps you cope with life's stressors so you don't give into the temptation to overeat. And exercise is the perfect prescription for hormonal times in your life such as PMS or menopause when you need "something" to take away your edginess, irritability, and cravings.

Have you ever wondered why all the men in your life seem to lose weight quickly, while it takes you forever to drop a pound or two? It's because men have so much more muscle mass, which helps them burn calories faster, so they lose weight easier than women do. And men don't have to deal with PMS or other hormonal changes

 SCREENING FOR COLON CANCER

It is recommended by the Centers for Disease Control and Prevention (CDC) that people should begin regular colorectal cancer screenings at age 50. Your doctor may want to do an earlier screening if you have a family member with early-onset colon cancer. Several colorectal cancer screening tests are available, including the following, but your doctor will determine which is right for you:

▶ **Colonoscopy:** a tube inserted into your colon that allows your doctor to examine the inside of your intestine.

▶ **Barium enema:** an X-ray of your intestine enhanced by inserting a contrast material (barium) into the colon through the anus.

▶ **Fecal occult blood test:** checks the stool for signs of gastrointestinal bleeding.

that may cause them to binge eat once a month. But with the fun cardio, strengthening, and slimming exercises in *Side Effect: Skinny*, you too can easily build muscle mass and experience quick and lasting weight loss.

Studies show that your basal metabolic rate accounts for about 60 to 75 percent of the calories you burn daily. Two other factors also determine how many calories you burn daily: thermogenesis and physical activity.

THERMOGENESIS (FOOD PROCESSING). About 10 percent of the calories you ingest each day are used for digesting, transporting, and storing the food you eat.

PHYSICAL ACTIVITY AND EXERCISE. The rest of the calories your body burns are determined by your physical activity and exercise (jogging, biking, dancing, playing with your kids, walking the dog, housekeeping, gardening, or team sports).

If you are inactive, you can only guess how inefficient your body is at burning calories. I want to help you challenge your body to get super efficient and blast that fat.

Along with aging, some common health conditions such as hypothyroidism may affect your metabolism. Your thyroid helps set your metabolism—how your body gets energy from the foods you eat. Hypothyroidism is an underactive thyroid gland and is increasingly common in women over age 60. But your doctor can order a simple lab test to detect hypothyroidism, and treatment is usually safe and effective.

 MUSCLE IS A METABOLISM BOOSTER

Fat burns 2 calories per pound while muscle at rest burns 6 to 10 calories per pound. When in motion, muscles burn up to 15 to 20 calories per pound. So my toning-up exercises are fabulous metabolism boosters that will help you blitz off the pounds.

10 DRUGS THAT CAN CAUSE WEIGHT GAIN

Here are 10 drugs that are known to have weight gain as a side effect. If you think one of these is stalling your weight loss, it warrants a conversation with your doctor. But I want to warn you: before you make any changes to your prescription drug regimen, you must consult with your physician. It's smart to evaluate your drug routine every few months with your doctor anyway, to make sure they're still right for you. As you lose weight on this plan, your prescription needs might change. But stopping a drug without discussing it with your doctor is dangerous business, so don't go down that road.

▶ Prednisone to treat asthma or inflammatory arthritis

▶ Prevacid to treat heartburn

▶ Nexium for heartburn

▶ Zyprexa to treat psychosis

▶ Paxil to treat depression

▶ Inderal to treat high blood pressure

▶ Lexapro to treat depression

▶ Depakote to treat seizures or mood swings of bipolar disorder

▶ Prozac to treat depression

▶ Diabeta to treat diabetes

Also, doctors have explained to me that commonly used medications taken for depression, high blood pressure, heartburn, and even allergies can contribute to weight gain. According to the *Physicians' Desk Reference* (PDR), more than 100 prescription drugs may cause weight gain by lowering the body's metabolism and allowing fewer calories to be burned and more to be stored as fat. Pretty shocking, right?

You wouldn't think that one little pill could hinder your weight-loss efforts.

Now the picture is becoming clear: even when you are trying your hardest to stay on a diet, various factors can work against you to slow down your metabolism and stop your body from burning fat. Let's put all of these scary statistics away for now because I have found some surprisingly easy ways to increase your metabolic rate—no matter what your age or diet history. In doing so, you can easily get past that weight-loss plateau, blast the fat, and get healthier, too.

IMAGINE THIS

Right now, imagine that you're wearing a large, bulky coat that weighs about 20 pounds. I want you to think about how this heavy coat affects every part of your life—from the way you walk, sit, and sleep to your activity level at home and at work. You will move slower, have difficulty

 WEIGHT OR BMI?

When I was a kid, the doctor's height/weight chart was the go-to resource to verify a healthy weight. Today, doctors use other measures to assess a patient's weight, including the body mass index (BMI). BMI is a number calculated from a person's weight and height. The BMI number correlates to your risk of serious health problems like hypertension, diabetes, high LDL cholesterol, and even cancer. The higher your BMI, the greater your risk of getting these health conditions. According to the Centers for Disease Control and Prevention (CDC), people with a higher percentage of body fat tend to have a higher BMI than those who have a greater percentage of muscle. It is the excess body fat—not muscle—that increases your risk of health problems. You can find out your BMI by using any of the online calculators available today. But remember—we're all built differently. While your girlfriend may be the same height as you, yet weigh 10 pounds more, both of you may be at your optimal weight, depending on certain variables such as age, bone structure, and genetics.

climbing stairs without getting out of breath, and feel hot, tired, and uncomfortable all the time. Now, imagine that you take off the coat. Can you feel the tremendous relief without the added weight on your joints, muscles, and heart? It's a huge difference; and that's how I want you to feel as you shed pounds on this program. Take note of the changes you experience: less pain, more energy, increased stamina, and a happier outlook.

No matter what your weight, no matter what your age, no matter what your blood pressure or cholesterol or blood glucose levels, I know that you can get healthier, move faster, and have more energy quickly as you kick-start your metabolism and lose weight, following the program in *Side-Effect: Skinny*.

I want you to get really serious about your health, so that you can live a long, happy, and productive life. I know that if you put yourself first, you will have enough energy and good health to be active and care for everyone around you. And if you make your health a top priority by losing the excess weight and reducing the risk of serious diseases, you'll get the best side effect of all: getting slim, trim, and fit. After all, that is how I define skinny—still feminine, but strong and toned, with curves in all the right places.

Look, I know it isn't easy to stay focused on your health when you are juggling responsibilities, caring for your family, and worrying about deadlines at work. But I also know that, no matter how busy

 DENISEOLOGY: WHAT YOU CAN CHANGE

There are so many things we cannot change in life, but we can change:

1. The way we eat

2. The way we move

3. The way we think

you are, you can lose those extra pounds and get healthier again. So throw away the past. Forget about those other attempts. Today is a new day—this is a fresh start. You have a perfectly clean slate, and you're ready to do the work, because guess what? The decisions you make right now, today, will make a profound difference in your health, your looks, and how you feel about yourself. Make a new, lasting commitment to your health, your body, and your future right now. Come with me on this journey; you'll be so glad you did.

CHAPTER 2

LOSE WEIGHT 7 DAYS AT A TIME

The beginning of a new season, month, or year symbolizes a fresh start. Even the beginning of a new week can start you on the right track…let's take it 7 days at a time!

—*Denise*

L et's get down to business. I wrote *Side Effect: Skinny* to be your healthy prescription for *life*, not just a temporary solution for a weight problem. You will start with Skinny Strategy 1: The 7-Day Fat-Blast Diet. Then the other 6 Skinny Strategies can be incorporated into your daily lifestyle, with each strategy building on the previous one to help you lose weight, trim your tummy, and get healthy quickly without resorting to fad, deprivation diets that only set you up for failure.

Now here's the really good news. What if I told you that you have permission to cheat—yes, cheat—on this diet? It's true. Every 7 days you can—no, you *must*—take time off from the 7-Day Fat-Blast Diet to have a decadent meal. How does homemade lasagna with a seven-layer salad, a slice of warm garlic bread, and ½ a cup of frozen yogurt sound? Or what about 2 medium slices of pizza with your choice of meat and veggies, a side salad, and a light beer? Maybe you'd like to have dinner out with friends and enjoy sushi, miso soup, and salad with sliced avocado and grilled salmon…and don't forget a glass of your favorite wine!

All of these dinner choices and more are yours on the 7-Day Fat-Blast Diet. I want you to plan your dinner dates, birthday parties, receptions, and cocktail hours around your weekly Super Splurge without the fear of regaining the weight you have lost. I know you have been on diets before and are tired of being deprived. Planning for your Super Splurge will give you even more incentive to follow my diet. (More on the Super Splurge in Skinny Strategy #3.)

CALORIE CONFUSION

My 7-Day Fat-Blast Diet is based on Calorie Confusion, which simply means varying your calorie intake every 2 days to trick your body into keeping your metabolism super-charged.

Here's why you will benefit with Calorie Confusion. Studies show that your body gets accustomed to the number of calories you eat daily. For example, if you eat 1600 calories every day for several weeks, your body gets used to this amount and your weight stabilizes. But what if you eat just 1100 calories a day for several weeks? Shouldn't you drop pounds quickly as long as you stay on a very low-calorie diet? Nope! While you may drop pounds initially on an 1100-calorie diet, over time, your body gets used to this amount and your weight will stabilize—the scales will not budge. Your body is pretty smart and it goes into starvation mode. It wants to hold on to the fat because it's afraid you're not going to give it enough nutrients to survive. And then, when you decide to eat more than 1100 calories, you will begin to gain weight even if you eat only 1400 calories per day, which is still a low-calorie diet. It sounds crazy, but that's how your body works. This weight gain happens frequently to women who live for months or even years on a semi-starvation diet of iceberg lettuce and carrot sticks, and then wonder why they gain weight when they add a slice or two of whole-grain bread to their meal plan. The bottom line is that, not only do starvation diets not work, they also cause your metabolism to slow down, making it nearly impossible to drop weight.

SHORT-TERM, LOW-CALORIE PLAN JUST FOR WOMEN

Side Effect: Skinny is a short term, low-calorie diet plan just for women. It is based on the latest scientific, dietary principles that promote health and wellness. In the beginning, for the first 3 weeks, I am recommending low-calorie menus so you will really see results in a hurry. But this isn't forever—it's only to give you a jumpstart.

However, during this time, if you're having any unusual symptoms like headaches, dizziness, or extreme hunger, or if you want a slower weight loss, I encourage you to eat more than what is recommended. Add an extra slice of whole-grain bread, a piece of fruit, or a yogurt or green smoothie. While your weight loss will likely be slower if you deviate from the diet, if you still follow the *Side Effect: Skinny* principles, you will be on your way to permanent weight loss and vibrant health. As with any diet and exercise plan, have a discussion with your doctor before you begin. And if you're pregnant or breast-feeding, put this book down for now—it's never a good idea to start a diet program during those special times in your life.

Here's a tip: In the diet world, it has been documented that people under-report the amount of calories they take in and over report the amount of calories they burn. In other words, we don't realize how many calories we're actually eating (or how many calories certain foods really have), and we think we're burning more calories during daily life than we actually are. This fact encouraged me to plan low-calorie, extremely nutrient dense menus that can be the basis of any healthy weight-reduction diet. *Nutrient dense* means you get the most bang for your buck. You get foods with the highest vitamins and minerals for fewer calories. You get lean protein instead of high-fat, high-calorie protein. And you get good, healthy, low-calorie carbs instead of simple carbs that are high in sugar, fat, and calories and won't satisfy your hunger pangs.

I want you to see results, so there are no more excuses why you cannot lose those last 10 or 20 pounds that have been haunting you forever. This plan will help you do just that.

IS THIS DIET SAFE?

Yes! While there are many unsafe ways to lose weight quickly (and I don't recommend those, nor will they keep that weight off), *Side Effect: Skinny* incorporates foods that pack a huge nutritional punch. The menus I have presented are high in antioxidants, phytonutrients, vitamins, and minerals, not to mention protein, carbohydrates, and healthy fats. This is a short-term diet that leads to long-term healthy eating.

When you follow the recommendations in *Side Effect: Skinny*, you are learning basic principles that not only help you lose weight but, more importantly, help you keep it off forever. You will find over the course of three weeks that food is almost secondary to the real principles that help you keep weight off.

What are the underlying principles of *Side Effect: Skinny*? Glad you asked. Here we go:

HOW TO SHOP. This includes which foods to put in the cart and which to leave on the shelf; which foods to keep and which to toss in the garbage.

HOW TO CHOP. You'll be eating a lot of whole foods on this diet, and that means you'll be doing quite a bit of choppin', slicin', and dicin'! This can be fun; I promise. You'll get to experience what it takes to prepare simple, healthful meals. If you're not so sharp with the knife (get it?), then consider another chopping device—there are lots of safe, easy-to-use ones on the market.

HOW TO DEVELOP YOUR OWN DIET PHILOSOPHY. You need to have a diet philosophy that you believe in to lose weight and maintain the weight loss. *Side Effect: Skinny* gives you a dietary philosophy that keeps you motivated so you can stick to your plan. I want you to believe in you and stay with this diet plan because you want the very best for you.

Weight loss doesn't happen overnight. (Sorry about that!) You need to work with the diet and truly make it yours. Following *Side Effect: Skinny* gives you the time you need to adjust so you can enjoy success.

THE 7 SKINNY STRATEGIES

Here are overviews of the 7 Skinny Strategies you will follow in this diet and fitness plan:

Skinny Strategy #1: The 7-Day Fat-Blast Diet

There are two levels of my 7-Day Fat-Blast Diet. They focus on different aspects of weight loss, including kick-starting your weight loss during the 3 weeks of Level 1, losing up to 10 pounds in those 3 weeks, and then blasting the fat as long as you need to lose weight with Level 2. As you reach your goal weight, you'll learn how to add favorite, healthy foods to the diet to stabilize weight loss.

The 7-Day Fat-Blast Diet is based on 7-day cycles. Every 2 days, you will alternate your calorie count, which will boost your metabolism. It's easy to stay on a diet when you know you can have more calories in a day or two. I encourage my friends to look forward to the higher-calorie menus and especially the weekly Super Splurge. Knowing that you can eat your favorite meal once a week makes it so much easier to stick with the diet every day.

Most importantly, if you follow my program and just take it 7 days at a time, your body will burn those unwanted calories and blast that fat, and you will look sexier and slimmer, lose that dangerous belly fat and get healthier too.

Skinny Strategy #2: The Fat Blaster Workout

This scientifically based exercise plan revolves around my own Interval Walking program, along with total body toning exercises I call 7-Minute Slimmers that you can do anytime at home or at the office. I will also teach you 3 simple stretches that you can do every morning when you wake up to get your body in a calorie-burning mode. You'll incorporate workouts into your daily plan, and I've built them into the daily program, so you'll have daily reminders to get your body moving.

My Interval Walking program is unique because it creates Muscle Confusion. This means that, because your muscles accommodate a specific type of stress over time, you must constantly vary your exercise frequency, intensity, and time (FIT) to avoid a plateau. Using the exercises in this strategy, you can create Muscle Confusion every day and keep your metabolism working at its peak.

The 7-Minute Slimmers will tone every muscle of your body from head to toe. These special strengthening exercises are extremely effective for women because you use 2 groups of muscles at the same time. You'll shape your abdominal muscles while toning your buttocks, or chisel your biceps while trimming your waist. I'm so passionate about exercise because it can lead to weight loss, lowering blood pressure and LDL cholesterol, managing blood glucose levels, preventing cancer, building stronger bones, boosting your mood, and more. That is why I believe that this exercise workout is so vital if you want to lose weight, keep it off, and get stronger, too.

Skinny Strategy #3: Super Splurge!

Why do women give up on diets? Because they don't have a strategy for overcoming cravings. They feel deprived at parties, miss having desserts with friends, and crave comfort foods like brownies, cookies, and cake. I believe that life is too short to be overly restrictive with eating. Besides, what do you do when cravings overwhelm you? If you are like most women, you give in and binge-eat. I do not want you to resort to binge-eating—ever.

With my 7-Day Fat-Blast Diet, you will look forward to "cheating" with a Super Splurge every 7 days to ease cravings associated with dieting. In this strategy, I will give you some fabulous and delicious ideas for the most-craved snacks and desserts, including lists of Super Splurge sweets. I'll also show you how to enjoy your Super Splurge, but still keep the calorie count to around 1500 calories on that 1 day. You will eat a light breakfast and lunch and then enjoy your favorite restaurant meal and cocktail. Also, you can switch your Super Splurge day if you know you are going out on a Saturday night—plan your week ahead and you can have the splurge of your life! You will factor your Super Splurge into your entire day's calorie intake.

Skinny Strategy #4: Lose Weight the Fast Way

Do you always snack while watching TV at the end of a long day? Millions of Americans admit to nighttime eating and drinking. The problem is that nighttime eating can set you up for weight gain. Not only do people tend to eat higher-calorie foods (and drinks) for snacks, but most of these people are also inactive, spending time sitting or lying down while watching TV. Honestly, there is a reason it is called "break-fast"—and if you aren't fasting at night, you cannot break it in the morning with a filling and enjoyable breakfast. In this strategy, I will ask you to eat only during the daytime for 12 hours—from 7 a.m. to 7 p.m.—and then your kitchen officially closes after dinner. I'll explain the latest theories on nighttime fasting, too, and how this will help boost weight loss.

Skinny Strategy #5: Top 14 Side Effect: Skinny Foods

This might sound crazy, but there are some powerful foods you can eat to boost the health of certain body organs…and these foods actually *look* like the organ or body system they help. You'll be amazed how a walnut, which looks like a brain, can actually improve your brain function, or the connection between blood-red beets and the health of your blood stream. Of course, you probably know the connection between carrot slices and eye health—but I'm giving you a visual reminder of why you should choose these foods for the health of your body and all its organs. I've incorporated these foods into the meal plans to make it super simple for you.

Skinny Strategy #6: Double-Your-Metabolism Foods

This strategy will give you the ultimate skinny on healing foods that are known to boost metabolism. I'll reveal the latest findings on apples and how they boost metabolic rate. Remember the grapefruit diet that helped you drop weight quickly several years ago? Well, scientists now realize that grapefruits actually *do* have fat-blasting power—and could dramatically reduce the size of your waistline. I'll give you cutting-edge information on many other foods such as green tea, certain dairy products, and green coffee extract that may help you reach your weight-loss goal faster and also boost your health along the way. Of course, most of these foods are also included in the meal plans and recipes, but I want you to really understand why you're eating them and what they do for your body.

Skinny Strategy #7: Daily Body Blitz

As you will learn in the last strategy, the most effective way to lose weight and keep it off is to keep your body active—daily—moving every chance you get and keeping your cardiovascular system in optimal health. With this last strategy, I will help you redefine daily exercise to include foot-tapping, dancing, stretching, pacing, jogging, and other enjoyable activities you can do 1 minute at a time any time of the day or night—even while talking on the cell phone, working at your computer, or sitting in rush hour traffic. I call these 1-minute exercises the Daily Body Blitz. When you combine this Daily Body Blitz with the other strategies, you will slash calories and boost weight loss and good health.

NOW YOU'RE READY TO GO!

Now that you understand the basics of the 7 Skinny Strategies, I'll bet you're ready to dive in. We're almost there. On each day of this program, I want you to remember that excellent health is the key to staying active and alert all your life—and it's the key to a long life, too. This program is designed, first and foremost, to help you improve your overall health. The foods and exercises in the plan can bolster your energy and improve your overall bodily functions. And who doesn't love a side effect of getting slim and trim?

Maybe you feel like you've heard all this before. You've tried every diet known to man, only to be disappointed time and again as the weight initially lost quickly finds its way back to your hips, waist, and thighs. Or maybe you gave up on other plans because you felt deprived, hungry, tired, or you just didn't see a difference on the scale. Maybe those diets were too restrictive or required you to purchase pre-packaged shakes, bars, or meals, which cost a fortune and left you feeling ravenous all day long. There's a better way.

The 7 Skinny Strategies in this plan will let you in on the very best secrets I've learned over the years for speeding up your metabolism and burning fat. There are no gimmicks, no special foods you have to eat, no complicated exercise moves you can't do, and no deprivation. Instead, you'll find simple meal plans, workouts you can easily incorporate into your lifestyle, and endless options and recipe ideas. You'll learn vital details about what makes your body lose fat and gain sexy muscle tone. I'm redefining the word *skinny*. Now when you think of the word *skinny*, instead of picturing bony, frail, or scrawny, I want you to think of strong, toned, and sexy, with healthy curves. That image you have in your head right now—that can be you!

I know you're ready to see amazing results, so let's get started. The first step is to dedicate yourself to the plan for just 7 days. After

 MEASURE YOUR WAIST...AND YOUR HEALTH

An easy way to predict your chance of heart disease is a test you can do yourself in the privacy of your own home. Take a measuring tape and wrap it around your waist. Stand tall and keep the tape measure flat and level with your belly button. Here are the safe measurements for women and men:

Women: 35 or fewer inches around

Men: 40 or fewer inches around

If you don't like the number you get, don't lose hope. You have taken a healthy step in the right direction by starting the 7-Day Fat-Blast Diet and Workout. Just keep at it, and you will be thrilled with your results—I guarantee it!

the first week, you'll have so much weight-loss success that you'll feel incredibly motivated to keep on going. Regardless of your age or physical fitness level, I know you can be strong and sexy. And I will be right here with you every step of the way while you're blasting away fat and laying the groundwork for a healthy life.

First things first. How can you know where you're going if you don't know where you're starting? Here are a few steps to help define your starting point and make sure you're organized and ready to go.

1. **Weigh yourself,** and write it here: _____. Make sure you weigh yourself without clothes at the same time of day, preferably early in the morning before you eat or drink. Weigh yourself again on Day 3 and then every other day after that. Write down your weight on the chart on page 212.

   I believe that weighing every other day is a positive reality check, whether or not you are dieting. Weighing yourself frequently keeps you highly motivated to stick with the program. Sure, some days the scale may not budge; other times the scale may show that you gained a pound or 2. But keeping an accurate and written account of your weight will let you see your progress over time and also help you tweak your diet and exercise program if you are not losing fast enough.

2. **Measure your waist,** and write it here: _____.

   You will measure your waist every 7 days, for as long as you follow this program. You'll find a space to write down your waist measurement in the Skinny Food and Exercise Log. Measure your waist without clothes on, at the same time of day, preferably before you eat.

3. **Talk to your doctor.** If you haven't been active for a while, make an appointment with your primary care doctor. You might need a physical examination to make sure you are in good enough shape to start this program. This is especially important for people over 50 and those who have diabetes, hypertension, asthma, a heart condition, or joint problems.

If you have questions about your health, now is a good time to write them down and ask your doctor for answers. If you have undiagnosed pain, be sure to talk with your doctor about this so you do not risk injuring yourself with the Fat-Blast Workout. If you take medication that causes your heart rate to either slow down or speed up, or if you take medication for blood pressure, type 2 diabetes, or other health conditions, ask your doctor how to do the exercises safely.

While you are seeing your doctor, put all your medications and natural dietary supplements in a little brown bag and take this to the appointment. Each medication may have side effects or contraindications that go along with it, so make sure to explore your medications in depth. Ask your doctor if these medications or supplements affect your heart rate in any way. Talking this through with your doctor is important so you can make sure to exercise safely, and I want to make sure you stay healthy from start to finish as you blast the fat.

 MARGO'S HEALTHY MAKEOVER

Margo, a 49-year-old accountant, wanted to lose 15 pounds to reach her goal weight of 130. She was positive that she followed the 7-Day Fat-Blast Diet to a T. However, I looked at her Skinny Food and Exercise Log after 5 weeks and instead of staying with the recommended Calorie Confusion menus, she was averaging around 2500 calories a day. When I showed her the real calorie calculations, Margo saw "in writing" where she had overeaten. She promised to carefully keep track of the foods and portions she ate and to continue her Fat Blaster Workout. I saw Margo a month later, and she'd dropped the 15 pounds and felt wonderful. The benefits of a slimmer waistline, more energy, and normal blood pressure gave her the incentive she needed to stay with the 7-Day Fat-Blast Diet and be forever fit.

Trust me, the 7-Day Fat-Blast Diet works. But you have to be honest and accountable by keeping track of your activity and calories.

SET SKINNY GOALS

You cannot measure your success in life without setting goals. If your goal is to lose 5 to 20 pounds or more with *Side Effect: Skinny*, then dieting and working out will help you achieve this goal. I'd like you to post your goal on a sticky note somewhere that you can see it, such as on the refrigerator. That way, you can be reminded of your weight-loss goal daily. Besides, others will see your goal and they can remind you and help you to be accountable. In fact, ask family members to crack the whip (gently) if they notice that you're skipping the gym one too many times. Or better yet, ask them to join you on your morning jogs. If you're supporting one another, everyone wins. But don't set yourself up for failure by not being realistic about your goals. You might want to set your goals in increments. Focus on the first 5 pounds and make that your goal. Once you achieve the simple goal, then set another goal to lose another 5 pounds. I know this is like taking baby steps, but it is very effective for staying focused and reaching your weight-loss goals.

4. **Keep a daily log of your exercise regimen and the foods and beverages you consume in the Skinny Food and Exercise Log** (page 212). It is easy to underestimate how much you are really eating. That's why it's so important to record everything you eat, and every exercise you do in the Skinny Food and Exercise Log at the end of the book. This will help you be more accountable and stay on track. People who journal about their food and exercise are usually more successful at their weight-loss efforts than people who don't journal. I want you to be successful, so if it goes in your mouth, it goes in the log.

5. **Gather the right exercise equipment.**

    - **Shoes.** A pair of cross-trainers are ideal for the different stretching, strengthening, and cardio routines you'll be doing on my Fat Blast Workout. A solid pair of sneakers with shock-resistant soles is perfect for hitting the ground walking or following my DVDs inside. The moment you lace up your walking shoes, you're instantly in the workout frame of mind.

- **Yoga mat.** A yoga mat is good to have for the slimming and stretching exercises you'll do in the Fat Blaster Workout. This rubber mat should be lightweight and small enough to store at home when you aren't exercising.

- **Dumbbells.** Weight training will help rev up your metabolism (and burn major calories!) with my 7-Minute Slimmers—my special strengthening exercises that burn twice the calories in half the time. Start with 3- or 5-pound weights to work those muscles harder and to tone those arms quicker. You can find Denise Austin Dumbbells at Rite-Aid drugstores across the nation.

- **Pedometer and/or heart rate monitor.** Pedometers allow you to count your steps and track your progress; you can even find pedometers, watches, and heart rate monitors wrapped all in one. Get one you can easily use, and keep it with you every day.

6. **Get comfortable clothes.** Go ahead and treat yourself to at least one new training outfit. Even if you exercise in the privacy of your home, I believe it feels better to wear attractive and movable workout clothes because it puts you in the mood to work out. Be sure to buy breathable fabrics, especially if it is warm outside, because you will certainly sweat on the Fat Blast Workout. When the temps cool down, you will want to layer your workout clothes, so you can take your sweats off as your body gets warmed up. Also, I recommend wearing a supportive sports bra for comfort and better back support, especially if you are larger-breasted.

WORK WITH YOUR FAMILY

If you're a mom, try getting up half an hour earlier to have "me time" while the kids are still asleep. That's what I do! Or if your kids rise and shine early, then look for a gym that has childcare or a kid's club. Also, you can push that stroller for your daily workout. I remember spending many hours pushing my babies and toddlers around the neighborhood to let them get fresh air and to give me a great body-trimming workout. If you have older kids, let them know that mom needs more "me time" to plan healthy menus for the family and to exercise. It is important to be a healthy role model to your children so this time apart is healthy. Ask your spouse or partner to help more with the household responsibilities so you have time to focus on your weight loss.

7. **Clean out your kitchen pantry and refrigerator.** Get rid of all highly processed foods, foods high in sodium (salt or MSG), and foods high in bad fats, sugar, and white flour. I always tell people that if you look at the nutritional facts on the package and don't understand the ingredients, then toss it in the garbage.

The best way to know you have safe and healthful foods in your pantry and refrigerator is to purchase whole foods or foods that are unprocessed and unrefined as much as possible, such as fresh fruits and vegetables, whole grains, legumes, fresh lean meats and fish, eggs, soy, and low-fat dairy.

Here's a good tip: if you see salt, sugar, or fat listed first on the nutritional facts label, you can probably toss that food, because it will not be too healthy. Here are a few bad foods to toss in the garbage:

- Boxed high-sugar cereal

- Potato chips, candy, and crackers (whole-grain crackers and air-popped popcorn are "safe")

- Cookies

- Pretzels

- Soda

- Sugar

- Sugar-laden fruit juice

- White flour

8. **Go shopping.** After reading through the 7 Skinny Strate-gies, make a grocery list of foods you will need for the diet. I have provided a sample shopping list at the end of the book on page 208, so you can copy this list and add to it with your favor-ite skinny foods, beverages, herbs, and spices.

9. **Check your attitude.** When you are on the path to creating a healthy lifestyle with *Side Effect: Skinny*, maintaining a posi-tive attitude is just as important as improving your eating habits and increasing your physical activity. I believe that being happy is vital to your success. If you find yourself thinking negative thoughts when you look in the mirror, I want you to imme-diately stop, look at yourself, and give yourself a compliment. Building up your self-esteem is vital to success on this plan. You have to believe you're worth the effort if you're going to have success. If you're in a bad mood and you want to skip your workout, stop and think. Going for a walk or doing a 7-Min-ute Slimmer can actually change your mood and make you feel better about yourself. Attitude is everything; and don't let out-side forces make your decisions for you. You hold the power to decide if you're going to be a go-getter or a quitter. No matter what, choose go-getter every time! You've already made a huge step by committing to this program—so keep the momentum going. Choose to exude confidence. Just think: In a few months, with your hard work and dedication you *will* be the healthy woman that people will look at and think, "Wow, I wish I had that trim body." You are on the right track, so keep up that pos-itive attitude.

10. **Ease your stress and chill each day.** Stress is terrible for your body and your weight-loss progress on *Side Effect: Skinny*. Chronic daily stress such as a ringing cell phone, screaming kids, barking dogs, or the constant notifications from the smartphone can add up fast, resulting in physical symptoms such as a faster heart rate or anxiety. Even worse, stress can lead to emotional eating, even when you aren't hungry, which adds up to one thing: weight gain. When you get stressed out, you may make bad health decisions such as grabbing a few cookies on your way out the door, skipping your exercise routine, or drinking alcohol at night to soothe your stressed-out state. It is important to adopt some healthy habits to improve your mood and well-being. As you get ready to start the 7-Day Fat-Blast Diet and Workout and the other Skinny Strategies, get pumped up—not stressed out! Make up your mind today to manage your stress level so you can stick with the 7-Day Fat-Blast Diet and get healthier for a lifetime.

11. **Make time for YOU.** Every day or, at a minimum, every week—do something for yourself and let family members and friends know that that time is yours and can't be rescheduled. I'm a firm believer in taking time out for you, and I don't believe it is being selfish. After giving to family, friends, and career, day after day, every woman needs to recharge her batteries, and that is okay. In fact, it will make you better at all of the various responsibilities in your life. Once you get into the habit of spending nonnegotiable time with yourself, you'll start to see a difference—in your figure, your health, and your mood. Many women who follow the 7 Skinny Strategies in *Side Effect: Skinny* find it challenging to carve out their own *alone* time. But I believe it's not a matter of how many hours in the day there are—I think it's a matter of priorities. If you find it hard to make "you" time, it's because you're putting something or someone else above YOU in the list of priorities. You might need to write down all those priorities and find a way to move yourself to the top.

MASTER THE 7 DIET "DOS"

I can't wait for you to be the fit and fabulous person you want to be—and you *will* be. Now that you're creating a healthier you, follow these tips to avoid common diet pitfalls:

1. **Eat Until You're Satisfied.** Believe it or not, if you want to lose weight, it is important to eat. Skipping meals can leave you feeling weak and hungry, which leads straight to overeating. Eat when you need to, but make sure you limit yourself to nutritious, strength-building foods.

2. **Include a Variety of Foods.** You've heard of diets that focus on one food, or that exclude whole categories of food from your life. Go for balance instead. Sweets, pasta, and breads have a place in your eating plan. The key is moderation. Make healthy foods the foundation of your meals.

3. **Quench Your Thirst.** Water helps you burn calories, boosts your metabolism, and fills you up. How's that for multitasking? Bottoms up, ladies.

4. **Concentrate on Your Health.** Diet pills, crash-dieting, and products that promise instant results are never a good idea. A slow, steady, balanced weight-loss plan like mine is the most effective and the safest. You'll feel great, and you'll protect your health too.

5. **Make it a Team Effort.** Staying motivated is so imperative. Find an exercise buddy in your neighborhood or at your office, ask a friend or family member to help you stay on track, or take advantage of my amazing online community.

6. **Get Moving.** If you're already eating healthy, exercise can tone muscle and give you lots of energy. Even just a few minutes a day can make a huge difference. Give it a try.

7. **Put YOU at the Top of your Daily To-Do List.** Shift your priorities so that you can make time for yourself, without feeling guilty.

JUST 7 DAYS TO SKINNY

If you can commit to 1 week—just 7 days—I promise you'll be on your way to losing all the excess weight and improving your health with better blood pressure, cholesterol numbers, blood glucose levels, and more.

Of course, I am hoping you'll stick with the 7-Day Fat-Blast Diet and Workout longer than just 1 week. I really think you'll love my plan and make a full commitment to the 7-Day Fat-Blast Diet once and for all, as you finally lose the extra pounds, burn that belly fat, and increase your lifespan, all while you begin to enjoy optimal health.

Millions of my fans and website visitors have successfully integrated my 7-Day Fat-Blast Diet and Workout into their busy lifestyles and have lost from 10 to 40 pounds—or more. Most of the women that started my 7-Day Fat-Blast Diet saw a weight loss of at least 7 pounds during the first 2 weeks and up to 10 pounds in 3 weeks! This is exciting news. As these women hit their goal weight, they all noticed a direct correlation with an improvement in their health, such as drops in blood pressure, LDL cholesterol levels, triglyceride levels, fasting blood glucose levels, and a decrease in chronic back, joint, and muscle pain. Truly, getting healthier is the best news of all.

CHAPTER 3

SKINNY STRATEGY #1:
THE 7-DAY FAT-BLAST DIET

It's all about moderation—not elimination!

—Denise

First, congratulations on your smart decision to lose weight and get healthy once and for all! Now that you have made the initial commitment, you are probably wondering about Skinny Strategy #1.

You've probably realized by now that I don't believe in starving or using extreme measures with my 7-Day Fat-Blast Diet. Unlike most diet programs, very few foods are off limits in this program. Instead, with my diet, you'll have reasonable and delicious meal plans already designed for you (yes, the menus are planned ahead!). You can easily follow the menus without a great deal of preparation or effort.

As a health and fitness expert, I'll tell you up front that many quick weight-loss diets set you up for rapid weight gain when you are no longer able to live on an ultra-restrictive diet of low-carb bacon and eggs or green tea and wilted lettuce for days to weeks. That is why, after doing much research, and talking to the nation's smartest doctors and weight-loss experts, I carefully devised my simple 7-Day Fat-Blast Diet that will let you do the following:

- ▶ Commit to just 7 days at a time: C'mon, you can do anything for 7 days.

- Avoid weight-loss plateaus by changing your caloric intake every 2 days with Calorie Confusion to trick your metabolism.

- Quickly drop up to 10 pounds in 21 days as you kick-start your metabolism.

- Blast another 10 pounds or more over the next 28 days.

- Develop solid, healthy, eating habits with an "eating plan for life" as you move toward your weight-loss goal.

- Maintain your weight loss as you learn how to add favorite foods—even comfort foods—back into your diet plan.

- Get healthier—improve your blood pressure, cholesterol, triglycerides, blood glucose, and more—as you eat for optimal health with the amazing side effect of getting skinny.

 IS THE 7-DAY FAT-BLAST DIET SAFE FOR PREGNANT WOMEN?

Honestly, pregnant women should not be on weight-loss diet. Instead, your goal should be a healthy pregnancy. You reach that goal by eating the right foods, exercising daily, and listening to your body. Generally, while many women believe they need to "eat for 2," pregnant women need only 300 additional calories each day (fruits, vegetables, whole grains, low-fat dairy products, and lean meats), along with prenatal vitamins that provide additional nutrients, including iron. Both weight loss and excessive weight gain carry risks during pregnancy. Adequate weight gain depends on your age, height, and pre-pregnancy weight. It's normal to gain between 25 and 35 pounds during pregnancy. But you should talk openly with your doctor about the nutritional plan that is best for you and your developing baby. If you are healthy and have no obstetric or medical problems, you should be able to do mild to moderate exercises. It's best to talk to your doctor before starting any workout program to make sure it's safe for you. Here's the bottom line: during pregnancy, focus on maintaining your health (and the health of your baby), not on your weight.

In *Side Effect: Skinny*, you'll start with my 7-Day Fat-Blast Diet that lets you eat to feel full while still losing weight quickly by alternating your calorie intake every 2 days over a 7-day period.

Along with the diet, you will do the Fat Blast Workout (Skinny Strategy #2) with my energy-boosting Interval Walking program, 7-Minute Slimmers, and Do-It-Yourself Tummy Tuck, along with other daily strengthening and stretching exercises. I am positive that my 7-Day Fat-Blast Diet and Workout will rev up your metabolism and force it to work harder and more efficiently, so you can avoid plateaus and get slim again.

MODERATION—NOT ELIMINATION!

With my 7-Day Fat-Blast Diet, you won't have to stop eating carbs or meat, or even your favorite comfort foods. The 7-Day Fat-Blast Diet doesn't include diet shakes or diet pills that can make you feel sick or cranky. Instead, I want you to eat 3 delicious meals a day—and I insist that you eat every last morsel. (Yes, for once you can be part of the Clean Plate Club!) Better yet, I will encourage you to snack wisely between meals and cheat on Day 7 with the Super Splurge.

 DON'T LET "ALL YOU CAN EAT" FOOL YOU

In addition to delicious fresh fruits and veggies, all-you-can-eat salad bars often offer a number of non-healthy options, too! Watch out for macaroni, tuna, and pasta salads, because they contain loads of fat and calories, mostly from mayonnaise. Go for veggies and fruit or bean or cucumber salad instead. Also avoid croutons, cheese, fried onions, and creamy dressings. Stick with a basic salad made with fresh veggies, like tomatoes, fresh peppers, cucumber, and onion, and get the dressing on the side—preferably light vinaigrette. In addition, even bacon bits, nuts, and seeds can add up quickly. If you want something with more crunch than those fresh peppers on your plate, try just a small teaspoon of nuts or seeds.

On my 7-Day Fat-Blast Diet, you can expect to see daily menus that include my favorite recipes for smoothies, Flatbread Pizza, Crispy Kale, Vegetarian Chili, and White Corn Scramble (my absolute favorite omelet for breakfast or anytime). Sounds mouth-watering, doesn't it? If these recipes are not what you were expecting, it is probably because you were conditioned to think that all diets mean deprivation. In my opinion, that theory is archaic.

Here is something you should know about my 7-Day Fat-Blast Diet: This is exactly how I eat every day. I love delectable food that won't weigh me down, so I'm sharing my favorite foods and easiest recipes with you because I would never ask you to eat anything I wouldn't eat myself.

Just like you, I crave tasty, whole foods because I like to feel full. I like yummy comfort foods like warm peanut butter toast for breakfast, delicious 7-layer salad for lunch, and my fish tacos with guacamole and tortilla chips for dinner—all of which you'll have on this 7-day eating plan.

THE TRICK IS CALORIE CONFUSION

A host of studies confirms that varying the calorie count during a weight-loss diet helps to "confuse" the body and keeps the metabolism working at top speed.

To keep your body working hard at shedding those pounds, I want you to vary your caloric intake (Calorie Confusion) the first 3 weeks (Fat Blast) and rotate your calories for 7 days as follows:

2 days at approximately 1100 calories

2 days at approximately 1175 calories

2 days at approximately 1250 calories

1 Super Splurge day at approximately 1500

I have given you the estimated calorie count for each menu for 5 weeks. The first 3 weeks (Level 1) are lower in calories to allow for a Fat Blast, or jumpstart, to your weight loss. The next 2 weeks (Level 2) are a little higher in calories.

You will notice that the calorie count of each daily menu is slightly higher after the first 3 weeks on the diet. It's difficult to cut calories dramatically for a long period of time, so I have added more calories to Level 2. The additional daily calories may cause you to lose weight at a slower pace. Still, you should anticipate losing up to 10 pounds—or even more—while you stay on Level 2.

Once you have gone through the sample menus for 5 weeks (pages 167 to 182), I want you to go back and highlight your favorite menus to create your own personalized Level 2 Plan. The calorie count in Level 2 is slightly higher, so vary the calorie count of the menus for 7 days to include the following amounts for each week until you meet your weight goal:

Select 2 menus that are approximately 1100 calories

Select 2 menus that are around 1200 calories

Select 2 menus that are 1300 calories

Select 1 Super Splurge menu that is around 1500 calories total (this is the same Super Splurge each week)

 7 BEST SALAD STUFFERS

Chicken breast, turkey breast, cold-water fish, shrimp, scallops, low-fat cheese, eggs, beans

Raw seeds and nuts (watch portion size)

Fresh fruit

Avocado (watch portion size)

Artichoke hearts

Hearts of palm

Water chestnuts

7 BEST MEALS IN 7 MINUTES OR LESS!

Fish or Shrimp Tacos—220 calories

Bean Bowls—160 calories

Flatbread Pizza—280 calories

White Corn Scramble—110 calories

Jicama Salad—280 calories

Fat-Blast Green Energizer Smoothie—80 calories

Fat Blast Fruit Energizer Smoothie—120 calories

LEVEL 1 BOOSTS QUICK WEIGHT LOSS

Level 1 is short-term (just 3 weeks) to help boost quick weight loss—so be sure to look forward to your Super Splurge on Day 7 where you can eat the dinner or snack of your choice.

If you follow Level 1 to a T the first 3 weeks, you can expect to lose as much as 2 to 5 pounds the first week; up to 10 pounds or more over 3 weeks or 21 days. However, if you substitute other foods, or if you ignore the exercises in Skinny Strategy #2, you may not lose the weight as quickly. That is why it is so important that you follow the plan precisely and record all your food and beverages in the Skinny Food and Exercise Log (page 212).

LEVEL 2 FOR LONG-TERM WEIGHT LOSS

You will stay on Level 2 as long as you need to drop pounds. Just continue to follow the meal plans in this book and vary the calorie counts of the weekly menus as described on page 167; the pounds will fall off.

Now, before you do anything else, I want you to empty your pantry of the things you know are bad for you. I know it's not easy to throw food away, but if you keep it on your shelves, you're more likely to eat it in a moment of weakness. Then, I want you to copy down the 7-Day Fat-Blast Diet Shopping List on page 208, and go grocery shopping for the delicious, healthy foods you'll be eating from now on. Add foods that you enjoy to the shopping list. Again, this diet is not about deprivation.

I'm so excited that in just 7 days you'll already feel so much better and so much sexier. Now let's review the delicious menus as you take a step toward a healthier and skinnier YOU.

 SLIMMER WITH 7 EASY WAYS

1. Cut out 1 alcoholic beverage a day

2. Choose a lettuce wrap over a bun

3. Drink coffee without sugar, and with skim milk

5. Ditch sodas and sweetened beverages

6. Avoid fried foods

6. Use mustard instead of mayo

7. Eat low-fat dairy products

7 BEST WAYS TO CUT CRAVINGS

1. Eat breakfast

2. Carry snacks with you

3. Remember you can have a Super Splurge once a week

4. Eat healthy fats (olives, avocados, walnuts)

5. Keep a food diary

6. Exercise

7. Love the healthy food you eat

 ## 7 COLORS TO EAT EACH DAY

1. Red (tomatoes, raspberries, peppers)

1. Orange (oranges, sweet potatoes, carrots)

3. Dark green (kale, mustard greens, broccoli)

4. Purple (blueberries, grapes)

5. Yellow (squash, peppers)

6. Light green (cabbage, Brussels sprouts, peppers)

7. Brown (whole grains)

 ## COOK ONCE, EAT TWICE!

That is, when you are making something wonderful, double the recipe and freeze half for another meal. I do this all the time and trust me, no one in my house has ever complained!

OVERVIEW OF THE 7-DAY FAT-BLAST DIET

Level 1: 21 Days

Commitment: Kick-start your metabolism and boost quick weight loss with a 21-day diet based on Calorie Confusion. Don't forget to have a Super Splurge every 7 days!

Level 2: 7 days—Repeat as Long as You Need to Lose Weight

Commitment: Continue the Calorie Confusion as you trick your metabolism to boost fat loss. By changing the number of calories you eat every 2 days, your metabolism will stay super-charged and the pounds will drop fast. Still take time for your Super Splurge every 7 days so you don't feel deprived. Develop healthy eating habits as you reintroduce other whole foods you love into your diet and focus on the exercises and activities you enjoy.

Level 3: Forever Skinny (The Rest of Your Life)

MAINTAINING YOUR LOWER WEIGHT

In reality, it is always easier to lose weight than it is to maintain the lower weight. When you are following a diet plan you know what to do and what to eat, and you have structure. Once you get to your weight-loss goal, many women start slacking off. They may stop writing down their food intake, exercise a little less often, and add in a few more snacks and desserts. At first, the pounds don't start coming back. But in a month or so, you will start to see significant weight gain. To keep the pounds at bay, it is important to focus on the *Side Effect: Skinny* habits you embraced during this diet:

- ▶ Staying organized with your meal plans
- ▶ Eating the recommended snacks to curb your appetite

- ▶ Shopping for the planned menus and snacks

- ▶ Exercising regularly using Interval Walking and the other workouts in Skinny Strategy #2

Remember: without exercise, you will be unable to keep the weight off. You must commit to staying active or the pounds will reappear. No one can escape this fact.

It doesn't take much of a daily/weekly/monthly calorie increase to regain your weight. Once you reach your goal weight, I suggest that you begin to increase your daily calories by 100 calories every 3 or 4 weeks. Keep adding calories slowly until you've reached approximately 1500 to 1800 calories a day. Then make sure your weight is stable.

Some women might need only 1200–1400 calories a day to maintain a goal weight; others may need more. Your ideal weight is very personal, depending on your metabolism and level of exercise. It can also depend on how much you move in the course of your normal day. Are you sitting all day long or are you constantly on the go?

If you start gaining weight, you know that you are eating too many calories for weight maintenance. Before you eat something that you know is not on the *Side Effect: Skinny* plan, look at the calories and add them into your daily total. If you are not very active you will not need many more calories than the *Side Effect: Skinny* weight-loss menus. It does not take much to start gaining those pounds again. Constantly think about what you are doing. Mindless eating will sabotage your best efforts to maintain your weight. You have to want the weight loss and goal weight badly or you will easily slip back into old habits!

Staying focused on both your food intake and your calorie output is crucial to weight maintenance. You can do this. Even if you have lost weight and regained it many times, this time can be different and, as always, the power of success lies with you. *Side Effect: Skinny* has given you all the tools you need to successfully lose and then maintain your weight. It is up to you to take it on and make this a lifetime success story: your success story.

HOW MUCH WATER DO YOU REALLY NEED?

If you don't like drinking water, now is the time to learn how to love it. Proper hydration is so important to staying healthy. Because the body is made up mostly of water, it makes great sense to replenish it with fresh H_2O instead of sugary sodas or fruit juices. Also, did you know the brain can mistake thirst for hunger? It's true. So before you grab a high-calorie snack, try filling up with water. Then wait 20 minutes to see if you are still hungry. I'll bet your cravings disappear. So how much water do you really need? We've all heard we should aim to drink 8 cups of water each day. But if you consider that you will lose around 10 cups of water per day, under normal circumstances, and more if the temperature is hot or humid, then 8 cups doesn't seem like enough! Now that you're going to be working out regularly, you'll also need to drink more. Take my advice and drink up—it is H_2Ohhh so good for you! One tip: if you're having a hard time getting used to the taste of water, try adding a lemon or lime wedge, mint leaves, or even sliced cucumbers or strawberries for a hint of healthy flavor.

WHAT ABOUT VITAMIN SUPPLEMENTS?

Getting plenty of vitamins and minerals in your diet is crucial if you want to stay healthy. I like to get the vitamins I need by eating plenty of healthy whole grains, fresh fruits and veggies, and lean protein. But sometimes when I am really busy or traveling, it is just hard to do. That is when a supplement can help to boost your intake of necessary vitamins and minerals.

You may want to buy a complete multivitamin that has the basics such as vitamins A, C, and D, folic acid, and vitamin B12. Some multivitamins are geared for specific genders and life stages such as child-bearing women, women at menopause, or senior women. Consider a calcium supplement if you don't drink enough milk or eat enough dairy products. Also, if you don't eat salmon or other cold-water fish, you may want to take a fish oil supplement to get plenty of omega-3 fatty acids that are important for decreasing inflammation in the body. I also take a vitamin E supplement for my heart health. No matter what combination of vitamins and minerals you purchase, always remember to eat a wide variety of nutrient-packed foods. That is the best foundation for better health. And discuss any new vitamins or supplements with your doctor, especially if you're also on prescription drugs, because there could be contraindications.

 ## HOW'S YOUR SLEEP HYGIENE?

One of the greatest problems most women I know complain about is sleep—not enough sleep, early morning awakenings, difficulty going to sleep, hot sleep, painful sleep, noisy sleep, and the list goes on. The problem is that too little sleep plays a huge role in weight gain. The latest sleep studies confirm that two important hormones—ghrelin (the hunger hormone) and leptin (the hormone that tells you "I'm full") are regulated by sleep—or lack thereof. Here's how to make sleep work for you. Try to get 6–8 hours of sleep each night to boost leptin, which is a good thing when you are dieting. If you get less than 6 hours of sleep, the level of ghrelin increases in the body (you don't want too much of this hormone). Now, there are times in our lives when we don't have as much control over our sleep schedule as we'd like; just ask any new parent. If you can't get enough sleep each night due to children, you certainly don't need to beat yourself up. Just do the best you can. But if your sleep issues aren't kid-induced, it's worth talking to your doctor about it. And employ these easy tips to relax and sleep well throughout the night:

A.M. SUNSHINE. Seek out sunlight in the early morning each day, because your natural circadian rhythm, which regulates your sleep, benefits from natural light.

KEEP YOUR BEDROOM DARK AND QUIET. Use black-out shades, an eye mask, and ear plugs to shut out the world while your body sleeps.

FIND THE OFF SWITCH. Turn off the computers, tablets, televisions, and smartphones an hour before you go to bed. Studies show the artificial light coming from such devices can keep you awake and make it difficult to feel drowsy.

AVOID CAFFEINE AFTER NOON. Watch out for hidden sources of caffeine, such as medications, chocolate, and dessert drinks. Try green tea if you need a pick-me-up in the late afternoon because it contains only 20 mg of caffeine).

NO BOOZE BEFORE YOUR SNOOZE. Don't drink alcohol within 3 hours of bedtime. Alcohol keeps you from reaching the deep stages of sleep and dehydrates you, too. Many people who have cocktails after dinner complain of waking up in the middle of the night.

SLOW DOWN. Encourage everyone in your house (including yourself!) to start winding down at a reasonable hour by doing something relaxing, like reading a book, taking a bath, or having a warm mug of herbal tea. You'll feel so much better the next morning, and that will make it easier to follow my 7 Skinny Strategies.

THE SKINNY REWARDS ARE YOURS!

After staying on my 7-Day Fat-Blast Diet, Level 1 for just 1 week, you will feel incredible. The women who have tried this diet say they feel leaner, cleaner, and healthier, and their clothes start to feel looser.

After only 3 weeks on Level 1, you will look noticeably thinner. Family members and friends will comment that you look younger or ask if you have been getting better sleep or if you have been on vacation. I promise you can expect and enjoy compliments at this point.

Without the extra pounds, you will feel more energetic and productive, which sure helps when juggling kids, careers, or commitments. And because you have so much more energy, you will feel like being more active and getting more exercise, including strength training, stretching, and cardio activities like walking, biking, swimming, or active gardening.

After just 8 weeks on my 7-Day Fat-Blast Diet, you will feel better than you have felt in years—maybe even decades—and if you have stuck to the plan, you will be able to be as active as you want without feeling out of breath or having nagging knee or back pain. Once you have lost all the unwanted pounds, I want you to stay on my 7-Day Fat-Blast Diet, Forever Skinny for a lifetime, adding more foods and calories, as you can tolerate them, while you maintain your new, skinnier goal weight. After all, once you reach your new weight, you'll *never* want to return to being overweight with related health problems.

 DOES THE 7-DAY FAT-BLAST DIET WORK FOR DIABETICS?

First, if you're diabetic, be sure you discuss any changes to your diet and exercise routine with your physician. If you're diabetic and you count carbs to keep your glucose levels in check, then my 7-Day Fat-Blast Diet can be a great tool to use in conjunction with your doctor's recommendations. The nutritional information accompanies *every* recipe in the Fat Blaster diet, so you can easily find those that meet your carb goals, and tweak your food servings as needed (for example, maybe your body requires more protein, fewer carbs). If you are unsure what your specific dietetic needs are, or how to make the necessary changes, copy the recipes you'd like to try and ask your doctor or nutritional adviser to help you modify them. The next step is to enjoy all those delicious new meals!

CHAPTER 4

SKINNY STRATEGY #2: THE FAT-BLAST WORKOUT

*I want to help you wake up your metabolism
so it works for you...the best that it can!*

—Denise

How does a firm, flat, attractive tummy sound? Pretty good, right? It's within your grasp; it just takes a little discipline. Now that you are preparing for the 7-Day Fat-Blast Diet, you are ready to kick-start your metabolism and lose more weight—starting today. The first strategy is to get up and get moving. In the second strategy, we're going to walk, stretch, and strengthen the body in a fun, easy way that wakes up your metabolism so it starts to work for you—not against you.

We're going to shape up your body in just minutes a day with my Interval Walking program, 7-Minute Slimmers, Do-It-Yourself Tummy Tuck, and other great exercises that are guaranteed to get rid of unwanted fat so you get healthier and look younger, sexier, and slimmer again.

I like to think of my metabolism as my own personal trainer—always there supporting me, making me work harder and harder. That is why I take really good care of my body with plenty of exercise, healthy food, and sleep. My metabolism goes into overtime when I'm the healthiest, working hard day and night to help me burn calories and keep me trim.

If you are the "Energizer Bunny" type who constantly has tons of energy, your metabolism is already revved up and that's great. However, if you are like many women, your metabolism may be slow. You may feel sluggish and have unexplained weight gain even though your diet hasn't changed that much over the years. I know you can rev your metabolism up again, using the 7 Skinny Strategies in this book...I promise!

If it has been awhile since you have worked out (or if you are brand new to the concept of exercise), don't get overwhelmed by the idea of incorporating exercise into your life. I'm here with you, every step of the way. You can do this—just take it 7 days at a time. No excuses!

I will help you find the best moderate-intensity exercise that is right for you and that you will enjoy. For now, I would like you to get started with some physical activity, whether it is my invigorating Interval Walking program on page 64, the 7-Minute Slimmers on page 54, biking with your kids or grandkids, swimming at the YMCA, or active gardening. Whether you'd like to live longer to see your kids and grandkids grow up, or if you want to look super hot for your next high-school reunion, my Fat Blaster Workout is your answer. You MUST start now, get up, and move more!

DO YOU HAVE AN EXERCISE PHOBIA?

I have met so many women through the years who cringe when the word exercise is mentioned. Maybe you can relate to Claudia, a 35-year-old sales rep who twisted her ankle during a Latin dance class. Even though Claudia was a passionate athlete in high school, she developed a real phobia of exercise and physical activity, fearing she would reinjure her ankle. Claudia reasoned that being less active would guarantee she'd never have a problem again. Wrong. Today Claudia writes in an email that she has high blood pressure and chronic back pain—and both health conditions are attributed to her weight gain.

Or, perhaps you are like 42-year-old Susan, a preschool teacher and mom of three, who has been so busy taking care of kids and students that she has ignored taking care of herself. Now overweight and out of shape, Susan stopped exercising after her third pregnancy because she could not find the time, and exercise caused her to feel out of breath.

Over the years, Susan has gained 30 pounds, and was recently diagnosed with high LDL cholesterol and pre-diabetes. In addition, Susan's waistline grew from 26 inches at age 22 to 36 inches 2 decades later. That is a whopping 10 inches of extra belly fat. We know that women who have a waist measurement over 35 inches are at higher risk for cardiovascular disease, Alzheimer's disease, and metabolic diseases.

As much as Claudia and Susan probably didn't want to hear it, I gave them much-needed wake-up calls. Exercise was the only way they were going to reclaim their health. They had to take a leap (literally!) of faith, tie up those walking shoes, and get their butt in gear, even if it was just for a half hour, 4 days per week. And you know what? They did it. Both women lost more than 10 pounds the first 3 weeks of the Fat Blaster Workout. Not only did they lose inches from their waist, but their tummies no longer pooched out. Bye, bye, muffin top! They said their mood was better and they were more productive both at home and at work. Claudia and Susan, like so many women I have worked with in the past, went from exercise phobic to exercise enthusiasts, from sedentary to sexy, and I was thrilled.

A NATION OF DIET FAILURES

Recently when I was flying to a conference in Phoenix, Arizona, to serve on a panel about kids' health, I read a study that claimed two-thirds of all Americans say they are on a diet to improve their health. (Now that is what I like to hear!) Ironically, the study concluded that very few Americans have decreased in size—no matter what diet they tried. So, what went wrong? Americans are putting forth the effort but not reaping the benefits. I'll tell you why:

THEY UNDERESTIMATE THE CALORIES EATEN. I have realized that most people misjudge the number of calories they eat each day. Many people *think* they are staying on a 1200-calorie diet when, in fact, they eat well over 2000 calories daily. And as much as we try to eat low-carb or low-fat, counting calories is vital in blasting the pounds away. That is why writing down *everything* that you eat—including drinks and "bites" of food —can help increase self-awareness and pounds lost. I'll show you how to pay attention to serving sizes and stay accountable to what you eat each day with my Skinny Food and Exercise Log on page 211. It is not nearly as complicated or time-consuming as you might fear. Pretty soon, it will be second nature. You eat a bite of food; you write it down.

THEY OVERESTIMATE THE CALORIES BURNED. For most of us, it takes cutting back 500 calories a day to lose just 1 pound a week. If you try to do this through exercise, you will need to go for the burn and do relatively intense exercise for an hour a day. However, many visitors to my website usually "guess" how long they've exercised and believe they have worked long and hard—when, in fact, they've barely moved at all.

Through the years, I have found that a combination of calorie reduction and added exercise helps blast extra pounds. For instance, eating 250 calories less each day and burning 250 more calories with moderate exercise results in losing 1 pound a week. For a guaranteed fat blaster, I recommend walking 10,000 steps each day, using a clip-on pedometer to measure how many steps you take. In addition, I have found being accountable for exercise each day is the secret to losing weight and keeping it off. My Skinny Food and Exercise Log on page 211 will help you do just that.

 SOMETIMES LESS IS MORE

Did you know that working out 30 minutes a day is just as effective as working out for an hour? It is when it comes to weight loss. It's true, according to a study published in the *American Journal of Physiology*. Researchers concluded that working out for 30 minutes gave good results on the scale, and that is good enough for me.

THE FAT BLASTER WORKOUT

As you start Skinny Strategy #2—The Fat Blaster Workout—I will focus on the following best types of exercise that let you burn fat and kick-start your metabolism, even when you are sitting and watching TV!

Kick-Start with Stretching

Almost all women benefit from daily stretching. Studies show that stretching helps increase the muscle's elasticity and can increase how long and hard you exercise. Of course, stretching is a feel-good action—it comforts your body and releases muscle tension—but it also conditions your muscles for moving. The more flexible you become with stretching, the less likely you are to get injured—and you know what recovery time due to an injury can do to your waistline (or hips). Stretches also help work out the kinks in the muscles of your neck, back, arms, and legs, improving your posture and even making you look taller.

Stretching improves flexibility, an essential component of *functional fitness*—the ability to perform the activities of daily living. Functional fitness enables you to zip the back of a dress, reach for a book on a high shelf, or bend down and pick up your child or grandchild. Walking becomes easier, and your sense of balance will get better, too.

3 Kick-Start Stretches

Here are 3 stretches to get you started each day. They put you in the right mindset for the whole day, help boost your energy level, and jumpstart your metabolism. All three of these stretches are fabulous for your spine—and your spine is your lifeline, so keep the muscles surrounding it strong and flexible.

1. RISE AND SHINE. For this full-body stretch, you'll stand tall with your feet hip width apart and knees slightly bent. Inhale deeply as you reach your arms overhead. Feet firmly grounded, reach up through the crown of your head and fingertips as you lengthen your entire body. Exhale and release. Repeat 3 times.

2. SIDE BEND. Stand with good posture, and extend both arms overhead. Keeping your hips stationary, bend laterally to the right to stretch your left side. Then do the same to the left and stretch your right side. Repeat both sides. I love this side bend stretch, because it helps energize your back. This is a fabulous exercise for women who spend time working on computers each day. Teach it to your coworkers.

3. STANDING ROLL-DOWN, ROLL-UP. Stand with good posture, knees slightly bent. Tuck your chin to your chest and bend forward, scooping your abs up and in as you bend. Dangle your hands to the floor, relaxing your head and neck, and now imagine someone has placed a belt around your tummy and is pulling it up. Exhale and slowly roll up, keeping your abs scooping upward the entire time. Keep your knees soft, not locked. Repeat.

 ## DO-IT-YOURSELF (DIY) TUMMY TUCK

If you are like most women, you want to have a nice, toned tummy. It's the number one problem area women ask me about every single day! Whether you have belly fat left over from a pregnancy or the result of poor posture or sagging muscles, or even menopause, a chubby belly is both unattractive and unhealthy. You've got to reeducate your abdominal muscles daily to keep them toned and tight, and your tummy flat. Here's my quick and easy DIY tummy tuck that you can do any time of day—even while standing in line at the supermarket, in the carpool line, at the water cooler, or while cooking dinner for the family.

First, stand or sit tall with your shoulders back. Now tuck in your abs and contract and hold for 5 seconds. Then let the muscles relax and then tuck them in again for 5 seconds. Each 5-second isometric contraction is equal to one sit-up.

Remember, practice makes perfect abs. Do my DIY Tummy Tuck any time you think about it—day or night—and you'll notice a great improvement in your posture and abs in just a few weeks. Also, the more you do the DIY Tummy Tuck, the more you'll remember to do it. It will become a habit, just like brushing your teeth or combing your hair.

LAZY BONES JONES

If you're like many women today, you might spend a lot of time sitting in front of a screen—either your computer screen, checking email or working; or the TV, watching the news or sit-coms. Did you know that all that time you spend sitting is working against you? Many women are more likely to snack when sitting too. You burn more calories standing than you do sitting, so get up off your rear as often as possible. I challenge you with this Skinny Strategy to spend no more than 2 hours at the computer or TV each day for an entire week. I guarantee your weight will drop during this time. Once you've hit 2 hours, you have to shut down the computer and turn off the television, and you can't go back on until the next day. (If you don't use your TV or computer for 2 hours a day normally, then good for you; you have a head start, but that means you need to cut down to no more than 1 hour a day for the week.) Think you can do it? I know you can!

If you work at a computer, I can't ask you to stop your job! But you must be diligent in staying off the computer and TV at home—maybe aiming for just 30 to 60 minutes. Also, look for ways to cut down on your "zombie" time at work, too. This means you need to get up and move around throughout the day, at least once per hour. Talk to your co-workers, walk the stairs, stretch at your desk, and get outside during your lunch hour.

Remember when you said that you have no time to exercise in your busy day? Well, you'll be amazed at how much more time you'll have for yourself when you start cutting down on TV and computer time. You can do it!

To start, you can do the 3 Kick-Start Stretches before you start the Interval Walking, 7-Minute Slimmers, or anytime at all. Each stretch takes only 1 minute—so for just 3 minutes each day, you are well on your way to an energized, skinnier, and healthier YOU.

My stretching guidelines:

MOVE INTO EACH STRETCH SLOWLY. When you reach your maximum stretch, hold it. Don't jerk or bounce to increase the stretch; you could pull a muscle, and a pulled or torn muscle hurts.

HOLD EACH STRETCH FOR ABOUT 20 SECONDS. The longer you hold that stretch, the more your muscles relax.

BREATHE SLOWLY AND DEEPLY. In through your nose, out through your mouth. Deep breathing engenders focus and calm, and floods your cells with energizing oxygen.

Get Sexy with My 7-Minute Slimmers

I know...you wish you could wave a magic wand over your body and instantly lose weight and feel amazing. Don't we all? You're looking for the simple trick that will take you to your goal, pronto. Well, are you ready for this? Shhh...don't tell...but here's the secret (are you listening?)—it's muscle! That's right. Build more muscle and your body will naturally burn calories even when you are not working out. No kidding.

A major key to revving up your metabolism is muscle mass. The reason? Muscles demand more energy from your body than fat does; the more muscle you add to your body, the more calories you'll be burning throughout the day.

In fact, muscles at rest can give you double the calorie burn of fat. Depending on your activity level, the added burn could easily be 40 to 50 calories per day, according to some studies, and even more when you're working out.

Don't we all admire women with sculpted arms and shapely legs? Those sexy muscles look great in a sleeveless dress, but they also work around the clock to keep you strong, burn calories, and aid in losing weight.

My 7-Minute Slimmers are integrated workouts that keep your muscles flexible, strong, and less susceptible to injuries. When muscles are strong, you are able to perform everyday activities easier, and you will have greater endurance and energy that will make you feel even sexier! You can do my slimming resistance exercises right in the privacy of your own home. As long as the moving muscle has resistance, it will respond.

The 7-Minute Slimmers use more than 1 muscle group at a time, which burns more calories than only working a single muscle. These are compound moves that make your time more efficiently spent. 7-Minute Slimmers are functional and easy-to-learn strengthening exercises that allow you to tone your muscles, burn fat and calories, and increase leanness—all in a single 7-minute session.

Strengthening exercises boost your overall health too. According to the American Heart Association, strengthening exercises lower blood pressure and reduce cholesterol levels, which, in turn, reduce the risk of stroke and heart disease. Strengthening exercise is also important in the prevention of osteoporosis. It can also reduce the risk of age-related loss of muscle mass, reduced muscle strength, and reduced aerobic power.

 TAKE YOUR PICK!

Along with doing my 7-Minute Slimmers, I highly recommend the following for strengthening exercises. Pick your favorite and add it to your workout regimen.

- ► Workout machines
- ► Free weights (dumbbells)
- ► Cans of vegetables from the pantry
- ► Elastic bands/resistance tubes
- ► Water (swimming or movement)
- ► Stairs
- ► A step
- ► An uphill climb
- ► Your own body weight as you push against the floor, a wall, or other object

7-Minute Slimmers

To do the 7-Minute Slimmers, you will need 3- to 5-pound dumbbells.

My 7-minute Slimmers target and tone the entire body for a complete strengthening workout. My full-body integrated exercises will help you finish your workout in half the time.

Now, every second counts. The 7-Minute Slimmers are extremely effective as you use two groups of muscles at the same time, such as muscles in the thighs while shaping the shoulders or the abs while firming the arms.

Standing Exercises:

REAR LUNGE/BICEP CURL

Body Benefits: Gives you sexy arms, trim thighs, and firm buttocks

1. Stand with your feet shoulder width apart. Hold a dumbbell in each hand with your arms extended straight down by your sides, back straight, and abs pulled in.

 GREAT HIPS HOW-TO

There are lots of things you can do to tone your hips and thighs quickly. Lunges and squats are two of the best exercises. My favorites are walking lunges: walk, lunge down, walk, lunge down, and keep going across the room. Floor exercises—like leg lifts—and yoga moves are also great thigh toners. To focus on your inner thighs, try doing the plié exercises that are done in ballet. Stand with your feet wide, toes out, and then bend your knees and plié down. As you come back up, squeeze your inner thighs.

Also, my *Fit in a Flash 7-Minute Solutions* DVD features exercises for your hips, thighs, and buttocks; all the moves are standing exercises that slim the lower half. You may also want to try my *Shrink Your Five Fat Zones* DVD, which lets you customize your workout to target your entire body head-to-toe.

2. Step your left foot behind you about 3 feet. Then bend your right knee so it is at a 90-degree angle, with the left knee pointing down toward the floor. Make sure that your front knee does not go over your toes.

3. Simultaneously lift and curl the weight toward your shoulder for a bicep curl. Using mainly the heel of your front foot, push up and get back to standing position and repeat with right leg.

4. Alternate each leg repeatedly for 1 minute.

SQUAT/OVERHEAD PRESS

Body Benefits: Lifts your butt and firms thighs and also gives you those sexy arms and shoulders.

1. Stand with your feet a little wider than hip width apart, abs tight, back straight. Keep your knees slightly bent. Hold a dumbbell in each hand, with your elbows bent and place your weight near the front of your shoulders.

2. Squat down, sitting way back and keeping your body weight through your heels.

3. Exhale as you press the dumbbells over your head for an overhead press while simultaneously returning to standing position, keeping space beside your ears. Lower your weights to shoulder height.

4. Repeat for 1 minute.

DEADLIFT/ROW

Body Benefits: Shapes and trims back of thighs and strengthens your upper back muscles; bye, bye, back fat.

1. Stand nice and tall with your feet hip width apart, knees slightly bent. Hold a dumbbell in each hand with your arms straight down in front of your body.

2. Keeping your abs strong and back straight the whole time, slowly bend forward at your hips to lower the weights toward the floor with your hands directly under your shoulders.

3. For the row, bend your elbows as you pull your arms up along the sides of your body, turn your palms to face the ceiling, and try to bring your shoulder blades together. Then, lower weights back toward the floor.

4. Now, as you return to standing, squeeze your buttocks and thighs (it's the squeeze that really helps lift and shape your butt). Repeat for 1 minute.

Floor Exercises:

CHEST FLY/TOE TAP

Body Benefits: Firms and lifts your chest and flattens your belly, especially below the belly button.

1. Lie on your back, and elevate both feet in the air with your knees bent so your legs are at a 90-degree angle.

2. Hold the dumbbell in each hand with your arms straight above and in line with your chest. Your back should be flat and your tummy should be tight. Your neck never comes off the floor.

3. Inhale as you lower your arms out to the sides, keeping them slightly bent in an arc position, opening up your chest and

 AIM FOR AWESOME ABS!

Along with the stretches, strengthening exercises and Interval Walking in Skinny Strategy #2, be sure to do abdominal-building exercise at least 3 times a week, whether it is the ever-popular crunches or the core-building moves of Pilates. Put working out your abs on your to-do list. Not only will you be stronger, you'll enjoy the lean, sleek physique that goes along with fit abs.

lowering the dumbbells, almost to the floor. Exhale and press the dumbbells up again, keeping them in line with your chest.

4. Simultaneously, using your lower abdominals, with your abs tight and your back flat on the floor, tap your right toe to the floor, and then return it to 90 degrees. Alternate your legs continuously for 1 minute. Take this slowly—you don't want to rush this one.

BRIDGE/TRICEP EXTENSION

Body Benefits: Slims your hips, firms your buttocks, and zeroes in on the back of your arms. No more underarm flab.

1. Lie on your back with your knees bent, feet flat on the floor, hip width apart, and heels about 6 inches from your butt. Weights are in each hand, close to your ears and shoulders, with elbows facing up towards the ceiling.

2. Contract your back, abs, butt, and legs, lifting your hips off the floor and raising the dumbbells straight up over your chest. As you lift your butt up off the floor (bridge), your arms will be straight (tricep extension). Your body should form a straight line from your knees to your shoulders.

3. Hold, then lower your hips and dumbbells, and repeat for 1 minute.

 SHOULD I IGNORE PAIN WITH THE FAT BLAST WORKOUT?

Absolutely not. If you feel pain (other than typical muscle discomfort from exertion), stop exercising immediately. Apply RICE—rest, *ice*, compression, and *elevation*—if you think it is a joint injury or muscle sprain, strain, pull, or tear. If the pain persists more than 1 or 2 days, or if you think the injury may be something more serious, definitely consult your physician. And don't start any physical activity again without your doctor's okay. Remember, looking after yourself is the priority.

BICYCLE

Body Benefits: Works all of the core muscles. Trims and slims your obliques—the sides of your waistline.

1. Lie on your back with your knees bent above your hips and your feet lifted so that your shins are parallel to the floor. Press your navel toward your spine. Place your hands behind your head and rest your head in your hands, keeping your neck and shoulders relaxed.

2. Exhale as you bring your right knee in toward your chest and rotate your left elbow toward your knee. At the same time, extend your left leg out straight. Then bring your left knee in toward your right elbow and extend your right leg. Continue to alternate your legs back and forth, simulating riding a bicycle for 1 minute.

FULL PLANK/KNEE TO OPPOSITE ELBOW

Body Benefits: Lengthens the transverse abdominis muscle—the most important muscle that helps keep your tummy flat. Also, it works your arms, chest, and shoulders.

1. Position your body in a full plank (or pushup position), balancing on your toes and palms, and zip up your abs.

 WHITTLE YOUR MIDDLE WITH HIP CIRCLES

Stand with your feet slightly wider than your hips. Soften your knees, allowing a very slight bend. Extend your arms at shoulder height from your sides. Firm your tummy and circle your hips, starting by sticking your left hip out to the left as far as you can.

Try to use only your tummy muscles to bring your hips in a circle, pressing your buttocks back and then your hips to the right, and then front. Do a Tummy Circle for 30 seconds in this counterclockwise direction. Then switch direction and circle for another 30 seconds. Think of this exercise like hula hooping, which also helps slim the waistline.

2. Keep your abs pulled in, back straight, and head extended so that your body forms one long line from the top of your head to your toes.

3. Contract and engage your abs as you bend your right leg, bringing the right knee toward your left elbow, while keeping your back as flat as possible. Straighten the leg, and then bring your left knee toward your right elbow. Keep your belly button pulled inward while continuing to balance on the palms of your hands.

4. Alternate legs for 45 seconds and finish with 7 pushups.

7 Tips for Exercising Outdoors

Exercising in the great outdoors is one of my favorite things to do, and I highly recommend it. It is a fabulous change of pace that will get your blood pumping and your senses engaged, and you'll soak up all that fresh air and vitamin D from the sun. You will also get in touch with your surroundings, and maybe learn your way around a park you have never visited or an unfamiliar part of town. In addition, outdoor workouts are free—no gym memberships or class fees to worry about!

To make the most of your outdoor workout:

▶ Dress for the elements. Wear a hat and jacket if it is cool outside.

▶ Drink plenty of water before you start and after you finish. If you are going to work out for more than 30 minutes, carry a water bottle with you or stop for a drink during the workout.

▶ Dress in layers, peeling them off as you warm up.

▶ Wear reflective gear if you exercise before the sun rises or after it sets.

▶ Bring music—you can carry an iPod with headphones—to keep you pumped up. Or, if you can, bring a friend.

- ► Wear sunscreen and sunglasses to avoid sun damage. I apply sunscreen first thing every morning right after I brush my teeth. It's a good habit to have as you can get sun damage even on cloudy, cold days.

- ► Wear supportive shoes. Whether you have running shoes or enclosed, leather shoes, you need a shoe that supports your feet and protects you from objects that can cut your foot. Avoid sandals and flip flops when working out.

Go on—take your workout on the open road. You'll be glad you did.

 THE POWER OF VITAMIN D

While vitamin D is commonly known to build stronger bones and boost immune function, did you know that it might also help with weight loss? Studies reveal that most of us don't get enough vitamin D and people who are overweight or obese may be at greater risk of low levels of this vitamin. The reason is that body fat holds onto vitamin D and makes it unavailable to the body.

Findings reveal that lower levels of vitamin D in the body interfere with leptin. Leptin gives your brain a signal to stop eating. It is thought that overweight people spend less time in the sunlight (the best source of vitamin D) so this deprives them of the necessary levels of leptin to stop eating. How do you resolve this? Get outside and get moving, or turn to your diet to boost levels of vitamin D. Most people need around 400 IU of vitamin D per day. The easiest way to get your recommended dose is about 15 minutes of sunlight, but you can also find vitamin D in certain types of fish, such as herring, mackerel, salmon and tuna; some fish oils, such as halibut-liver oil and cod-liver oil; and foods fortified with vitamin D, such as milk and some cereals. If you cannot get the recommended amount from your diet or the sun, you should consider talking to your doctor about supplements.

Rev Up with Fat-Blasting Cardio

In addition to the stretching and strengthening exercises in the Fat Blaster Workout, I want you to add my 30-minute Interval Walking program to kick-start your metabolism. Cardio exercises are a great way to get in shape, burn calories, and lose weight. Also known as aerobic or cardiovascular exercise, cardio includes any type of exercise that gets your heart rate up. It's an absolutely vital part of your fitness program. My walking program increases heart rate and keeps it higher for a certain period of time. It helps your heart and muscles use oxygen more efficiently, and muscles that frequently receive oxygen-rich blood stay healthier. But remember with my Interval Walking or any new cardio exercise to always start slowly and increase gradually!

Interval Walking is the best exercise to boost your metabolism, because you are not walking at just one pace. This cardio exercise works because it fires different muscles, which causes Muscle Confusion. Because your muscles accommodate a specific type of stress over time, you have to continually vary your exercise *frequency, intensity,* and *time* (FIT) to avoid a dreaded exercise plateau. Using Interval Walking, you can fire different muscles, create Muscle Confusion and keep your metabolism working at its optimal level.

Not only does cardio exercise help you to blast the fat and allow you to maintain a normal weight, it also helps your heart and muscles to work efficiently. Did you know your heart is also a muscle? So you need to condition it just like you do your biceps. By conditioning the heart you're also

 TRIM YOUR THIGHS ON THE PHONE

If you spend a lot of time on the phone, like I do, don't just sit there—make it a workout by "pretending" to sit! Here's how: Lean your back lightly against a wall, making sure to press your spine flat. Slowly lower your body along the wall until your knees are bent to at least a 45-degree angle, but no more than 90 degrees. The motion should feel like you are lowering yourself into a chair. Hold for as long as you can, up to 60 seconds. Repeat.

helping fight heart disease—the number one killer of women. By staying active throughout your day, you can go from flab to fit at any age!

Cardio/aerobic exercises boost the amount of oxygen delivered to your heart and muscles, which allows them to work longer. The best part about cardio is that your metabolism stays charged for up to 2 hours after your workout ends, so you'll continue to burn fat and calories even after you have stopped exercising. In that way, cardio is like a gift to your body that keeps on giving—and you definitely deserve it.

On a side note, daily lifestyle activities such as sweeping the floor, carrying groceries from the car to your home, pushing a lawn mower, or active gardening will improve your aerobic conditioning. Whatever raises your heart rate and keeps it up for a period of time will help you be aerobic as you rev up your metabolism and lose weight.

To Start Interval Walking

You'll love this heart-pumping, core-sculpting, total-body workout. Interval Walking is one of the most efficient and effective workout routines I have ever designed, and you can do it anytime, anywhere.

I recommend that you wear comfortable clothes and a good pair of walking shoes for Interval Walking. You'll also need a watch or clock nearby so you can change intervals as discussed on page 66.

You can do Interval Walking indoors or outside, but I believe that walking out-of-doors lets you benefit from extra vitamin D from the sun. Besides the vitamin D, researchers at the United Kingdom's University of Essex revealed that exercising out-of-doors boosts self-esteem and improves overall well-being. Still, if you choose to exercise indoors, you'll need a 6-by-6-foot square of space, or a treadmill.

Rate Your Fat-Blast Workout on a Scale of 1–7

Before I give you the Interval Walking instructions, I want to help you understand how to rate your Fat-Blast Workout, so you know how you should feel during the different exercise intervals. This is important to be sure you are revving up the metabolism and not walking at a snail's pace.

I devised the following 7-point rating scale to help you assess how much you must work during exercise. Using the Fat-Blast Workout Scale, you can determine if your workout pace is a 1 (very light), a 4 (moderately strong), or a 7 (peak fitness zone; a nice clip!)—or anywhere in-between.

1 = Very light (Just warming up)

2 = Moderate (Starting to enter the work zone; heart is beating faster)

3 = Somewhat strong (You can still talk easily, but you feel your heart pumping)

4 = Moderately strong (You are working hard; heart rate is higher)

5 = Very strong (Your heart is beating fast)—FAT-BLASTING ZONE

6 = Near fitness zone (You are breathing a little more quickly)—FAT-BLASTING ZONE

7 = Peak fitness zone (You are almost breathless; it may not be as easy to speak, but you're moving at a nice clip!)—FAT-BLASTING ZONE

As you do the Interval Walking, you will want to push yourself at certain times to enter the Fat-Blasting Zone and then pull back slightly to catch your breath again. Looking at the scale, you can determine how hard you should work at each 2- and 5-minute interval. My husband Jeff does the same interval workout on his stationary bike and finds it really effective—enough to break a sweat. In addition, my workout DVD *Sculpt and Burn Body Blitz* offers a similar interval workout, if you'd like an alternate routine.

To Do: Interval Walking—
30 Minutes at Least 4 Times a Week

Preparation: You'll need comfortable clothes, good walking shoes, and a watch or clock to time the 2- and 5-minute intervals. Or do what I do—put a playlist together with a mix of 2-minute and 5-minute songs for the full 30-minute walk!

FIND THE BEST TIME

The best time to exercise is whatever time best suits your schedule. I work out in the morning so I don't have to worry all day about how I'm going to squeeze in a workout. Too many times I say, "I'm going to do it later," and it never gets done. Physiologically, it doesn't matter when you do it as long as you do it. Research has found that the morning or daytime tends to work best for women who have family commitments around dinnertime. In addition, many women who exercise late in the evening have difficulty falling asleep because their bodies and minds are keyed up and stimulated from exercise. Find what works best for you and stay with this time until it becomes a life habit.

Allow 30 minutes for this workout. You should do the Interval Walking at least 4 times a week, 30 minutes each time. If you choose to do it more frequently, you may lose pounds faster. You can alternate Interval Walking with Interval Biking, using the same 2- and 5-minute intervals to pump it up and blast the fat. Or, do the same Interval Walking on a treadmill or elliptical to get a great fat blasting workout.

5 MINUTES Start by warming up, walking at a nice pace and pumping your arms. As you get close to 5 minutes, walk with purpose. Get your heart rate up to a 3 out of 7 on the Fat-Blast Workout Scale.

2 MINUTES The next 2 minutes, aim for a 5 out of 7 on the Fat-Blast Workout Scale to enter the Fat Blasting Zone. Give it all you have, pumping your arms back and forth and going as fast as you can walk for 2 minutes.

5 MINUTES You will take it up another notch from the first 5 minutes. At this point, you are picking up your pace, your blood is pumping, and your breathing is quickened. Again, aim for level 4 out of 7 on the rating scale.

2 MINUTES This is a big blast. Walk really fast for 2 minutes. Pump those arms. Move those legs! Push that body! If you can, bring it to a jog if your knees are healthy. Again, move up to a 6 out of 7 on the rating scale, as you are breathing more quickly now and you are fully in the Fat-Blasting Zone.

5 MINUTES You should continue to walk fast for 5 minutes, making sure you feel comfortable and can talk as you walk. You should be around 5 out of 7 on the Fat-Blast Workout Scale with your heart pumping hard.

2 MINUTES Another big fat blast for 2 minutes. Walk as fast as you can, or jog if you can. Push yourself to hit 6 out of 7 on the Fat-Blast Workout Scale.

5 MINUTES Continue to walk at a brisk pace, pumping your arms as you do so. Aim for a 5 out of 7 on the Fat-Blast Workout Scale.

2 MINUTES Now, keep blasting the fat as you pick up the pace to give it 100 percent. This last fat blast is a really fast clip—all the way to 6 out of 7 on the Fat-Blast Workout Scale. Change it up and jog if you can do it!

2 MINUTES Now slow down. Do arm circles as you walk slowly for 2 minutes. Cool down until you return to a level 1 or 2 out of 7 on the Fat-Blast Workout Scale. This cool down slowly brings your heart rate down gradually and allows you to ease back into your normal routine.

 EMPOWER YOURSELF!

I wrote *Side Effect: Skinny* to help you gain self-worth so you feel really good about yourself. I want you to believe that you are beautiful on the inside and out. When you feel empowered, you make better choices. You care about your health because you love your body. You make healthy decisions about exercise, what you eat, and how you spend your free time. Stay empowered for optimal health.

After this workout, you should stretch, so perform the 3 Kick-Start Stretches discussed on page 51.

Other Options

If you're not a walker, there are other options for cardio exercise, it just depends on what you like to do. While the Interval Walking will boost your metabolism fast, other cardio exercises for getting in shape include running, jogging, biking, the elliptical machine, step aerobics, dancing, swimming, cross-country skiing, and so on. Mix it up, so you don't get bored. The key is to make sure you get your heart rate up while exercising, and to do cardio regularly. And of course, have fun.

 TRAIN LIKE YOU LIVE

I believe that your workout should mirror your everyday life. You work hard for a while and then lay back some. You push harder some days and then move slower other days.

READY, SET, GO!

As you start the Fat Blaster Workout, I want you to focus on just 3 minutes of stretching each day, using the stretches on page 51. In addition, I want you to do Interval Walking or other cardio exercise (biking, swimming, jogging, tennis) at least 4 days each week, 30 minutes each time. My Interval Walking program burns calories fast and you can do it anytime, anywhere—even while watching TV!

You will focus on the 7-Minute Slimmers the alternating 2 days or anytime you want to strengthen your body. In addition, do the Do-it-Yourself Tummy Tuck all day long—anytime you are standing or sitting and can hold the tuck for 30 seconds or longer.

I have listed the exercise schedule in the 35 days of menus—either Stretches and Interval Walking or Stretches and 7-Minute Slimmers each day for 6 days. Always do more if you can—I strive to exercise for 30 minutes a day. On Day 7—Super Splurge, I want you to have a great time playing with family and friends, but stay active!

SAMPLE EXERCISE SCHEDULE:

Day 1: Stretches and Interval Walking

Day 2: Stretches and 7-Minute Slimmers

Day 3: Stretches and Interval Walking

Day 4: Stretches and 7-Minute Slimmers

Day 5: Stretches and Interval Walking

Day 6: Stretches and Interval Walking

Day 7: Day Off and Super Splurge!

7 TIPS TO GET STARTED

Here are 7 tips to help you get started with the Fat-Blast Workout:

1. Make up your mind; it is now or never!

2. Block off time on your daily to-do list for the Fat-Blast Workout. Do not allow anyone to come between you and your workout—set this as a priority.

3. Unplug your telephone or turn off your cell phone so you will not be interrupted.

4. Find a place in your home that is quiet and roomy so you can stretch and strengthen without bumping into furniture.

5. Wear a workout outfit that makes you feel attractive. It helps to psych you up, and puts you in the mood to move around more! You are worth the investment, believe me.

6. Do your exercises at the same time each day so the Fat-Blast Workout becomes a habit, just like brushing your teeth or hair.

7. Split up the exercises into smaller time segments if you find yourself too busy to exercise. Even doing a little bit of exercise for 10 minutes at a time, 3 times a day, is helpful for losing weight and blasting the fat.

EXERCISE WITH A FRIEND

Through all my 30 years in the fitness business and talking to millions of people, I have found that those people who exercise with a friend, spouse, or significant other are far more successful than those who try to do this alone. Your exercise partner (your spouse, partner, friend, or family member) can serve as your motivator, and conscience. Besides

 7 MUST-HAVES FOR A HOME GYM

Many women prefer to exercise in the comfort of their own home. Exercising at home allows you the most flexibility for fitting a workout into your schedule. Plus, when you consider all the workout DVDs and home gym equipment, working out at home has never been easier, so you can't use the weather as a reason to skip a workout! Here are some basics you might consider including:

▶ Yoga or exercise mat

▶ 3- to 5-pound weights

▶ Balance and stability ball

▶ Resistance bands

▶ My workout DVds

▶ DVDs on beginning yoga, tai chi, and stretching exercises

▶ A mirror to check your form

that, talking with someone during exercise helps to pass the time in a fun way as you share stories and catch up on the latest news. Researchers from Indiana University's Department of Kinesiology revealed that spouses who worked out with their partners had a low quitting rate of 6.3 percent while spouses who worked out without their partners had a huge 43 percent quitting rate. Along with working out with a friend, you can inspire your friend or spouse to follow your example. Not only does it help you to maintain fitness, but it can also help them lose weight and get healthier. It's a win-win!

JOIN AN EXERCISE GROUP

You might also consider joining a fitness class at a local health club, YMCA, or school. Or check out a nearby mall, as most enclosed shopping centers sponsor early morning mall-walking groups. Some even have medical personnel who monitor blood pressure, do regular health screenings, or answer health questions.

NO MORE EXCUSES!

I have designed the workouts in this strategy to be fast and effective. If you are still overwhelmed by the idea of finding 30 free minutes most days to exercise, try making a few of these simple changes:

BE AN EARLY RISER Wake up half an hour earlier and get your workout out of the way first thing in the morning! Pop in a DVD

 KEEP ACCURATE RECORDS

Recording your exercise activities and times in the Skinny Food and Exercise Journal on page 211 is important for staying accountable to this program. Research shows that people who record the food they eat and their daily exercise are more successful with weight loss.

and get the blood pumping from the comfort of your living room—you don't even need to change out of your PJs.

NOT A MORNING PERSON? Try getting everything you'll need for the morning rush ready the night before, like preparing tomorrow's dinner or setting out lunches for the kids. That will buy you at least 30 minutes of time somewhere during the next day.

SPLIT IT UP If you can't fit in a single 30-minute activity period for the Interval Walking, break it into 10-minute brisk walks throughout your day—2 trips around the block of your office, or a walk to the park while pushing your child's stroller. Easy.

WORK IT IN Have a lot of shopping to get done this weekend? Get there early and promise yourself that you'll walk a few brisk laps of the entire mall before you start shopping. (Then treat yourself to a healthy lunch out!)

 NO TIME?

Many women complain of having no time to exercise, no matter how they try to rework their daily to-do list. Here are some great ways to sneak in some exercise that I use when I'm short on time:

- ▶ 10-minute walk before work

- ▶ 10-minute walk at the mall before you shop

- ▶ 10-minute ride on the stationary bike before lunch (or after work)

- ▶ 10-minute walk on your treadmill while kids nap, or during noon news

- ▶ 10-minute swim in your pool

- ▶ 10-minute bike ride with your spouse or child

- ▶ 10-minute walk around the block

- ▶ 10 minutes of low-impact aerobics using my DVDs

DANCE IT OUT Blast the stereo and dance around with your kids (or by yourself—no one's looking), do a few jumping jacks, lunges, or just shake your body while folding the laundry or doing any other chores. Music motivates you to get up and move—at least it sure does for me!

NEW TO WORKING OUT?

If this is brand new territory for you, start with indoor or power walking, light jogging, or even alternating between the two, until you get your body used to activity. Swimming and water aerobics are also fun and effective forms of cardio (and total-body toning), particularly if you have joint pain or knee issues, because the water provides resistance to the muscles, but doesn't cause painful impact from hard surface pounding. Don't worry about whether you are

 7 WAYS TO CHANGE IT UP

A great way to stay motivated or overcome a weight-loss plateau is to change up your routine with a new activity. Here are some great suggestions:

► Take a class in something you have always wanted to try such as dance, tai chi, or yoga.

► Ask an adventurous friend to plan a surprise activity or outing for both of you.

► Change the route of your regular walk to stimulate your mind with new scenery.

► Change the time of your Interval Walk. If you normally walk in the afternoon, set the alarm and walk early in the morning.

► Invite a friend to join you on the Interval Walk. Talking to someone can make the time fly by.

► Make short trips by bike or on foot instead of using the car.

swimsuit ready or not! Once you hop in the water, no one can see your body anyway.

KEEP MOVING!

I know it is hard to stay committed to any behavior change such as exercising daily. I also know how much better you'll feel if you exercise, stay fit, and eat right. Not only will you feel more alert and have more energy, but you'll be healthier too—and that's the ultimate goal!

Try to think of exercise as *movement* rather than a strict regimen. Make a list of some physical activities that you enjoy or would like to try, such as trail hiking, mountain biking, swimming, swing dancing, golf, and skiing. Guess what? Doing any of these things regularly will get you in shape.

In the meantime, do little things regularly to ensure that you reach your fitness goals. Take the stairs whenever you can; and when you're shopping, stroll the entire mall or shopping center at least once. Think about it. A 20-minute brisk walk around the entire mall burns up 150 calories. Do it twice! That is 300 calories, plus it is fun, and you get to window-shop and people-watch all at the same time. Be creative, find an exercise that you like, and do it.

Simply knowing how much better you will feel if you eat right and stay fit should be enough motivation for you to follow the 7-Day Fat-Blast Diet and Workout consistently. But if you need more motivation, consider taping pictures of your kids or grandkids to the bathroom mirror. Seeing these precious children and knowing you want to watch them grow up is great motivation to eat healthy and be active. Believe me, when you devote yourself to leading this lifestyle, you'll be healthier, happier, and more energetic. When you have those moments when you overeat, or days when you miss a workout, don't let it throw you off track. Return to your routine the very next day, and keep up the good work.

Of course, there are days when I overeat and don't exercise. I'm not perfect! Come on ladies, I'm human, too. I don't go around eating carrot sticks and running hours every day. If I have a slip-up and eat a sugar cookie (or two!), I don't harbor guilt about it, I forgive myself and I get back on track the next day. Just don't let it go too many days without getting back on track. Go out there and work out, because it is the workout that will keep you going.

CHAPTER 5

SKINNY STRATEGY #3: SUPER SPLURGE

You only live once. Why not live as healthfully and vibrantly as you can?

—Denise

"Sure, I could stay on a diet," Brittney said honestly, "if only I could eat hamburgers and French fries occasionally. I really do love fruits and vegetables, but also I crave fast food once in a while."

Sound familiar? Aren't we all like Brittney in that we do enjoy the healthy diet fare—fruits, vegetables, whole grains, lean protein, nuts and seeds, legumes, and low-fat dairy—but after a steady diet of this for a week, we crave something else…a splurge! Most of the time that splurge is fast food, a warm brownie, dinner at a favorite restaurant, party foods such as appetizers and alcoholic beverages, or other intense cravings.

Many of my girlfriends complain that they can't stay on diets long term because they get derailed by food cravings. They feel deprived at cocktail parties, miss eating dinner out with family and good friends, and drool at TV advertisements of scrumptious comfort foods like cobblers, cookies, and cake.

I believe that life is way too short to be overly restrictive with eating. And so many diets are so full of "no-no's" they take the joy out of eating. In fact, I tell women that once they reach their goal weight with

Level 2 of the 7-Day Fat-Blast Diet, they can eat 80 percent healthy food and 20 percent comfort food if they cautiously watch their weight and don't gain the extra pounds back. I believe food should be your friend—not your enemy. Learning how to have a healthy relationship with food—even favorite treats every now and then—is far healthier than prohibiting certain foods until you get major cravings and start to binge eat.

Side Effect: Skinny is a weight-loss book to help you get healthier and, oh yeah, skinnier. But while following my 7-Day Fat-Blast Diet, I want to give you some clear-cut guidance on how to manage your cravings by cheating once a week. Here's my rule for your Super Splurge:

ENJOY A SUPER SPLURGE EVERY 7 DAYS

Allowing a "cheat day" is a key strategy to staying compliant to the 7-Day Fat-Blast Diet. Knowing that you can really splurge and plan a dinner out with the family or have a cocktail and appetizers with good friends will keep you satisfied. However, if you suppress your cravings and restrict yourself to the low-calorie meal plan and never splurge, chances are great that you will binge on foods that cause you to regain your weight.

 ARE YOU GAWKING AT FOOD PORN?

Do you start to drool when you see decadent photos of unhealthy foods on the internet, in magazines, or on TV commercials? There is a reason for it. Studies show that when you see high-calorie foods, it triggers the appetite-control signal in the brain. When this control center is stimulated, it can lead to overeating, or even weight gain. Some studies show that just looking at food triggers a rise in ghrelin, the "hunger hormone" that increases appetite (and the one we want less of!). Also, marketing surveys report that pictures of desserts (not fruits and veggies) are most likely to be shared online. The message? Watch what you look at so you can get (and remain) healthy and trim.

On page 79, I will give you delicious ideas for your weekly Super Splurge, which is why I absolutely love *Side Effect: Skinny* for my friends, you, and myself. I have found that eating a luscious dinner at a favorite restaurant or having a delicious, calorie-laden dessert once a week helps to increase satiety and cut back on my cravings throughout the week.

LET'S BLAST THOSE CRAVINGS!

I know you have cravings; we all do. But dealing with stubborn food cravings when you are trying to lose weight can be more than just annoying—giving in can undo weeks of hard work and effort.

That is why I recommend staying full all day long with the 7-Day Fat-Blast Diet. Eating the filling and nutritious foods and snacks outlined in the 7-Day Fat-Blast Menu Plan (page 185) will help suppress ghrelin, the hunger hormone that triggers a ravaging appetite. Here are some tips to move past cravings without bingeing or racing off track.

STOP AND THINK! If you feel hunger coming on, you shouldn't automatically reach for food. Before you eat, take a minute to think about what you are feeling. Ask yourself if you are really hungry. If you haven't eaten in a while and your energy is low, maybe your

 AVOID FOODS HIGH IN SODIUM

Canned meats

Canned fish

Canned soups

Canned tomato products and juices

Canned vegetables

Frozen prepared meals

Processed meats

Salted snacks such as popcorn, chips, crackers, and pretzels body is telling you to eat. If that is the case, grab one of the snacks on page 83 and you'll feel better in no time.

ARE YOU THIRSTY? Thirst can also feel like hunger. Pour yourself a refreshing glass of water and then see how you feel. Add a squirt of lemon or lime juice or a few cucumber or orange slices to the water to heighten your senses.

USE DISTRACTION. If you have just eaten, you might be having a craving. One of the best ways to beat cravings is to distract yourself. Get outside and take a walk. Call a friend, play a game on your phone, or simply get up and move around to a different area of your office. I have found that simply changing your surroundings can change the way you feel and help beat that craving.

CHEW AWAY YOUR CRAVING! Here's another simple trick: If you are having a craving, pop a piece of gum in your mouth. Sometimes the act of chewing is enough to get your mind off that pesky craving. You can do it. (I avoid sugar-free gums and candies because they often contain sorbitol, a sugar substitute that can cause GI distress.)

 AVOID FOODS HIGH IN SIMPLE SUGARS

Cakes

Candy and gum

Canned fruits in syrup

Cookies

Frozen yogurt and sherbet

Fruit juice

Pies

Regular sodas

Sweetened drinks

EASE PMS SYMPTOMS

Most women with PMS experience symptoms such as irritability, sluggishness, mood swings, and food cravings during this time of the month. While there is no cure for symptoms of PMS, these nutritional and exercise solutions may help:

► Stay on the 7-Day Fat-Blast Diet because it is balanced with a variety of complex carbs (vegetables, grains, fruits) and a moderate amount of lean protein, legumes, and dairy.

► Exercise regularly—even during PMS—to reduce emotional stress and keep your body fit. Exercise may decrease PMS symptoms because of the rise of endorphins (the body's feel-good hormones). Also, regular cardio exercise helps to decrease fluid retention and is effective in boosting mood in women with mild depression.

► Avoid alcohol during PMS each month. Alcohol is a mood-altering drug that can compound feelings of anxiety and depression. Also, many women have a decreased tolerance for alcohol prior to their menstrual period and this may cause you to get intoxicated quickly.

► Avoid caffeine before and during your menstrual period. Caffeine can exacerbate PMS symptoms, worsening the sleeplessness and anxiety you feel.

► Reduce sodium and salt in your diet to lessen fluid retention. Sodium can lead to bloating, edema, and fluid weight gain during PMS. Reducing sodium can ease these symptoms.

► Add just a splash of lemon juice in your water for a natural diuretic.

► If you experience hypoglycemia or low blood sugar during PMS with symptoms of fatigue, dizziness, and the shakes, divide your meals on the 7-Day Fat-Blast Diet into 6 small mini-meals that are rich in complex carbs and protein and low in simple sugars.

MY 7 FAVORITE TENSION TAMERS

The next time you are feeling stressed out or overwhelmed, be sure to try 1 of my 7 favorite tension tamers to soothe your mind and get you back on track.

1. BECOME A BATHING BEAUTY. There is nothing like taking a hot shower or bath before you crawl into bed at night. It will help you unwind and leave that harmful stress behind. Add a few drops of lavender essential oil to a warm bath for deeper relaxation.

2. LEARN TO MEDITATE. Meditation is not as complicated as you might think. In fact, it can be as easy as breathing deeply, sitting alone in a quiet space, or following a guided meditation DVD or podcast. If you want to get serious about meditation, try taking a meditation class and learn more about breathing techniques and the benefits of clearing your mind.

3. SET A NIGHTLY TEATIME. Some people find that a hot cup of herbal tea relaxes them after a busy day. Chamomile and peppermint teas, in particular, are said to help relieve insomnia.

4. CLEAR OUT THE CLUTTER! Keeping your home clean and free of clutter is a key component to healthy living. Enlist the help of your spouse and kids to clear out junk and store stuff that is not being used. Coming home to a clean, organized, and clutter-free environment will give you one less thing to stress over.

5. PLAN A GIRLS' NIGHT OUT. Researchers say that women who maintain close ties with other women enjoy such health perks as lower blood pressure, increased immunity, and even a longer life expectancy. Get in the habit of catching up with the ladies in your life at least once a week—go for dinner, drinks, a dance class, a movie, or start a walking group together.

6. GET HELP. If your kids are young, consider hiring a babysitter for a couple of hours each week or propose a trade with a friend or neighbor who could babysit in exchange for another favor or errand.

TRY THESE 7 GUILT-FREE SPLURGES

I grew up in a big family, surrounded by lots and lots of food—including sweets. I believe it is okay to splurge once in a while, but I always try to eat better the next day. I know you will have days that you have cravings on the 7-Day Fat-Blast Diet, especially for chocolate during PMS. If so, consider these 7 Guilt-Free Splurges:

1. 2 Tootsie Rolls

2. A fat-free fudgesicle

3. A cup of hot chocolate with skim milk

4. ½ cup of fat-free chocolate pudding

5. ½ cup of nonfat chocolate milk

6. 2 chocolate kisses

7. 2 tablespoons of M&Ms

Once you hit your goal weight, *occasionally* go for a real chocolate bar. Or, for now, wait until your Super Splurge day and go for the rich chocolate-chip cookies, an ice-cream sundae, a chocolate milkshake, or homemade brownie.

TAKE YOUR FOCUS OFF FOOD

So many women come up to me at seminars and tell me that as soon as they start a new diet like my 7-Day Fat-Blast Diet, they are suddenly faced with more cravings than before. I think we all are that way—longing for what we know we shouldn't have. Still, when you take the focus of your life off food, it sometimes leaves behind a big (doughnut-shaped!) hole. That is because so much of life revolves around meals and eating—shopping, cooking, entertaining. In a given day, you might go to a restaurant for lunch, meet your sister for coffee (and cake), and then plan a special dinner for your kids.

But when you start a new diet, you no longer can eat all the goodies you'd normally buy or make. It's hard to know what to do with yourself. It's difficult to make homemade peach cobbler for the family but not have a piece yourself. When the aroma of peanut butter cookies fills the house, how can you not break down and eat 1...or 2? I feel your pain.

As you commit to my 7-Day Fat-Blast Diet, challenge yourself to include the entire family. For instance, instead of serving a favorite chocolate cake or blueberry pie, give the family bowls of fresh blueberries with a sprinkling of cinnamon on top. Opt for naturally sweet baked apples for dessert instead of apple cobbler. Offer baked Idaho potatoes instead of French fries for less fat and fewer calories. Your family can benefit from your new lifestyle and diet, and you'll all get healthy and trim.

Furthermore, it's OK if you bring fruit salad instead of layer cake to a family cookout, or a plate of cut-up veggies and some light dressing instead of mac and cheese to a party. You have the power to take charge of every situation, so wield that power. Your family will understand and support you—they might even thank you!

 ## SAVOR SOME CHOCOLATE

Enjoy a square of dark chocolate to rev up and bliss out! Indulge in 1 square and then close your eyes and let it melt in your mouth. The dark variety is rich in anandamide, a molecule which the researchers at the University of California, Irvine, have linked to the same euphoric state you feel following a good workout. Other stimulants found in dark chocolate are caffeine and theobromine.

COFFEE OR NOT?

While a cup of coffee certainly won't cause any harm, I recommend limiting your intake of caffeinated beverages—including certain teas and sodas—as much as possible. The caffeine found in these beverages can cause you to lose water, if consumed in large doses. So aim for no more than 2 servings a day.

NO TIME TO PREPARE? HERE ARE 7 EASY TIPS!

Here are some easy tips to avoid giving into daily cravings.

1. Look for quick-prep side items at the grocery store. For example, plain frozen veggies can be steamed in the microwave in less than 10 minutes, as can instant brown rice.

2. Buy bagged salads at the grocery store and add your favorite seasonal fruits such as sliced apples, strawberries, or blueberries. Toss a few walnuts in the salad for crunch, and you have "fast and delicious."

3. Get sliced bagged apples (sweet or tart) at the grocery store. These can be opened, rinsed, and served with a roasted chicken and packaged salad for a Fat-Blasting Meal-in-a-Minute!

4. Pick up some prepared foods from the deli counter, such as roasted turkey and rotisserie chicken (just stay away from the fatty skin and mayo-laden pasta salads).

5. Whip up a homemade veggie pizza in a jiffy. Simply spread low-sodium tomato sauce on a premade whole-wheat pizza crust, add some healthy toppings (such as broccoli, spinach, fresh tomatoes, black olives, and a sprinkling of Parmesan), and pop it in the oven for a few minutes!

6. When eating takeout is truly unavoidable (try not to let this happen more than once a week!), opt for healthier options, like

steamed shrimp and vegetables (with sauce on the side) from your local Chinese restaurant, a grilled chicken sandwich, or a single-patty hamburger minus the cheese on 1 slice of bread (open-face style) or on a large leaf of romaine lettuce from the neighborhood burger joint. Or try veggie-loaded grilled steak or chicken fajitas (without the fatty extras like sour cream) from the nearby Mexican chain.

7. Buy boil-in-a-bag rice. It takes only 10 minutes to prepare, and it even comes in whole-grain and brown varieties!

SUPER SPLURGE ON THE ROAD

Heading out of town? If you travel a lot, you know how tricky it can be to stick with your eating plan. But just because you're in a hotel or a restaurant doesn't mean you can't eat well. Follow these tips and you'll be good to go!

EAT AS YOU WOULD AT HOME. Control the size of your portions at each meal. Portion control can make—or break—your dieting efforts, especially with restaurants supersizing meals or fad diet plans that encourage unlimited amounts of protein or other foods.

 EXERCISE AND CRAVINGS

Findings show that eating before a workout (even if it's a short, 10-minute workout) can help suppress hunger pangs, so you're less likely to slip up later. Remember, exercise boosts your metabolism so you will burn calories throughout the day and so you may feel a bit hungrier, especially on the days you do the Interval Walking. Since you're working the calories off, you may be able to eat a snack on exercise days. I'm not telling you to splurge each day or over-eat, but I'm letting you know that if you keep your body fueled with healthy foods listed in this book, it will help you stay energized so you can work out even more and lose that extra weight.

If you cheat by miscalculating your serving sizes, you're only cheating yourself.

IF YOUR ORDER ARRIVES AND IT IS ENOUGH FOR 3 PEOPLE, ONLY EAT 1 SENSIBLE PORTION. If you have a fridge in your hotel room or are staying with friends, you can ask the waiter to box up the extras before you even start to eat so you won't be tempted—and you can enjoy the leftovers as a guilt-free meal on another day. Better yet, ask about portions when you order and then see if your friends want to share.

SNACK BEFORE YOU GO. If you know you'll be tempted by rich foods, have a healthy snack before dinner. You'll feel fuller and will be less likely to indulge once you arrive at the restaurant.

KNOW THE LINGO. Avoid menu items that are described using the words *au gratin, crispy, fried, tempura, alfredo, cheesy, buttery, butter sauce, crunchy, beer-battered, crusted, pan fried,* or *creamy.* These are the buzz words that signal major calories. Stick with choices that are baked, broiled, poached, or steamed instead. Now, those are some menu smarts!

SUBSTITUTE. If a dish comes with fries, don't hesitate to ask for it with a salad, baked potato, or a steamed veggie instead. Likewise, if a meat or veggie is prepared with lots of heavy oils, ask about lighter preparation options or choose another dish. Restaurants want to make you happy (you are the customer, after all), so chances are they'll be willing to help.

SHARE. If you are dining with a friend, split an entrée, an appetizer, or even a dessert! It is a simple way to cut calories and not feel deprived.

Don't dread the pounds you envision you'll gain on your next vacation or fall off the wagon on your next trip. By thinking ahead, you will be equipped to travel in *healthy* style!

7 LOW-CAL DAILY SNACKS

There are lots of low-calorie foods that are healthy snacks, if you think you need a splurge before Sunday! Of course, the first that come to mind are fruits and veggies—and because there are so many to choose from, you never have to worry about eating the same thing all the time. Realize you may not lose weight as quickly if you add snacks to your 7-Day Fat-Blast Diet. But other low-cal options include the following:

- ▶ Low-fat yogurt
- ▶ String cheese
- ▶ 1 hard-boiled egg
- ▶ A handful of pretzel sticks
- ▶ 3 cups of air-popped popcorn
- ▶ Baked tortilla chips with salsa
- ▶ ½ English muffin with a teaspoon of peanut butter

 SHRINK-WRAP YOUR SERVING SIZE

Keep these tips in mind to control your serving sizes.

- ▶ A cup of fruit should be no larger than your fist.
- ▶ 3 ounces of meat, fish, or poultry (a normal serving) is about the size of your palm or a deck of cards.
- ▶ 1 to 2 ounces of nuts equals your cupped hand.
- ▶ Serve your meal on salad plates and pack away the large dinner plates.
- ▶ Store snack foods in tiny sandwich bags so you are sure you are eating no more than 1 portion.
- ▶ Ask for a kid's meal or small size—not the supersize portion.

LADIES, (DRUM ROLL!)...IT IS TIME FOR THE SUPER SPLURGE!

The Super Splurge allows you to have a large snack or a large meal on Day 7 of the 7-Day Fat-Blast Diet—between 7 a.m. and 7 p.m. You may have anything you want on this day as long as you keep your TOTAL day's calorie count to 1500 or less. This allows you to have a very simple breakfast and skinny lunch, no snacks, and then your Super Splurge. It's super easy to follow. You'll see in the menu that I have provided suggestions for a light breakfast and a light lunch. The Super Splurge snack or dinner is all in your court. Determine what and where you want to eat ahead of time, make sure it does not exceed 1500 calories for the day, and then eat and enjoy! Many prepackaged sweets, chips, salsa, colas, and alcoholic beverages have the calorie count listed on the nutritional label (check serving sizes to make sure it is only 1 serving). With other homemade splurges (cookies, cakes, pies) it may be more difficult to accurately assess the calories. Also, before you eat at your favorite restaurant, look online to see if they have calorie information for their menu items so you can more easily keep track. Knowing what you're going to order in advance will help keep you focused on your healthy eating goals. If your craving is for salty foods like chips and dip, nachos and salsa, a small slice of pizza, or a glass of wine or 2, that's fine. Just tally up the total day's calories to make sure you are staying true to your diet.

SWEET SUPER SPLURGE SUGGESTIONS	
Nestle' Crunch—Fun Size 3 bars	210 calories
Peanut M&M's—Fun Pack 2 bags	80 calories
M&M's—Fun Pack 2 bags	180 calories
Snickers—Fun Size 2 bars	160 calories
Milky Way—Fun Size 2 bars	150 calories
Kit Kat—Fun Size 2 bars	100 calories

SWEET SUPER SPLURGE SUGGESTIONS

Hershey's Chocolate Bar—Fun Size 1 bar	90 calories
Reese's Peanut Butter Cup—1 cup	80 calories
Butterfinger—Fun Size 1 bar	100 calories
Twix—Fun Size 1 bar	80 calories
York Peppermint Patties—1 patty	70 calories
Twizzlers—1 treat size pkg	45 calories
Almond Joy—1 snack size bar	90 calories
Milk Duds—1 treat size box	40 calories
Butterfinger—1 snack size bar	100 calories
Milky Way—1 snack size bar	90 calories
SweetTARTS—1 treat size pkg	50 calories
Tootsie Pop—1 pop	60 calories
Tootsie Roll—1 small roll	13 calories
Activia Desserts—1 dessert	120 calories
Brownie—1 small serving	250 calories
Chocolate bar—1 standard size	281 calories
Chewy Chips Ahoy—1 cookie	120 calories
Chocolate chip cookie—1 cookie prepared from recipe	100 calories
CLIF Mojo Bar—1 bar	200 calories
Kashi TLC Oatmeal Dark Chocolate cookies—1 cookie	130 calories
Keebler Chips Deluxe Chocolate Lovers—1 cookie	80 calories
Krispy Kreme Chocolate Iced Glazed Doughnut—1 doughnut	240 calories
Luigi's Real Italian Ice—1 serving	100 calories
McDonald's Chocolate Chip Cookie—1 cookie	160 calories
McDonald's Fruit 'N Yogurt Parfait—1 parfait	150 calories
McDonald's Strawberry Sundae—1 sundae	280 calories

SWEET SUPER SPLURGE SUGGESTIONS	
McDonald's Vanilla Cone—1 cone	170 calories
Pepperidge Farm Milano Cookies—1 cookie	100 calories
Planters Fruit & Nut Trail Mix—1 serving	140 calories
Skinny Cow Chocolate with Fudge ice cream cone—1 cone	150 calories
Snack Pack chocolate pudding cup—1 serving	100 calories
Starbucks Cappuccino (2 percent milk)—12 ounces	90 calories
Starbucks mini doughnut—1 doughnut	130 calories
Starbucks Caramel Macchiato—12 ounces	180 calories
Starbucks Treat-Sized Double Chocolate Cookie—1 cookie	130 calories
Wendy's Junior Size Frosty—1 junior size	150 calories

EATING OUT SUPER SPLURGE

I believe that eating out is part of the fun in life! I love to meet my girlfriends for brunch and have family dinner out with my husband and daughters. But you must make skinny choices in the foods you select. I don't believe in restricting anything from your diet when you're using your Super Splurge, so you can enjoy yourself at any restaurant you want. But read the menu carefully. What you order will make all the difference, especially when you have a whole list of temptations at your fingertips!

 KNOW YOUR ITALIAN

Even on your Super Splurge day, menu items that say *fritto*, *saltimbocca*, *Alfredo*, or *carbonara* are all way too high in calories if you eat more than just a couple of bites. Instead, opt for lighter (and equally delicious) menu items that are described as *griglia*, *marinara*, and *puttanesca*.

HOW-TO SUPER SPLURGE GUIDE FOR RESTAURANTS

Here are some tips to keep in mind for your Super Splurge. Since your overall goal for the day is 1500 calories, but you still want to enjoy a decadent "cheat," it's important to find balance. If you walk into a restaurant ravenous and ready to gorge yourself, you'll likely exceed your 1500 calories in a single meal, never mind the entire day. These are tricks you can use to still enjoy the splurge, feel full, but not go overboard.

Mexican Restaurant

▶ **Choose corn instead of flour tortillas.** Corn tortillas are also a great replacement for fatty chips when it comes to scooping up the veggie-filled salsa.

▶ **Go for fajitas, not tacos.** Not only will you get lots of veggies, but you can choose the quantity of cheese and beans to add.

▶ **Substitute a side salad for rice.** Spanish rice is often fried before it's steamed, so you end up getting a lot more fat and calories than you may realize.

▶ **Go for skinny margaritas.** Regular margaritas will cost you about 300 calories. But ask for a skinny variety, made with tequila, lime juice, and a hint of agave nectar.

Asian Restaurant

▶ **Start with soup.** Almost all Asian soups are broth-based, so you don't have much to worry about.

▶ **Enjoy green tea.** Not only is it filled with antioxidants, but it will also keep you full so that you don't overeat.

▶ **Avoid fried items.** Spring rolls, tempura, and fried noodles should be avoided. Order steamed dumplings or summer rolls (wrapped in rice paper) instead.

- ▶ **Sauce on the side.** If you get the sauce mixed in, your food will be swimming in it. Getting it on the side allows you to use just enough to season your food.

- ▶ **Try chopsticks.** You'll eat more slowly than you would if you use a fork. The extra time it takes will allow you to get a true sense of fullness.

Italian Restaurant

- ▶ **Start with a salad.** Watch out for creamy dressings and Caesar salads, which have loads of fat.

- ▶ **Choose minestrone or vegetable soups**, which have fewer calories and fat than cream-based soups and pasta e fagioli!

- ▶ **Skip the bread basket.** Be especially careful of garlic bread or breadsticks, which are often smothered in butter.

- ▶ **Go red.** When it comes to sauces, choose marinara, red clam, or puttanesca sauces over cream-based or Alfredo sauces.

- ▶ **Skip the side dish of pasta.** Ask the waiter for a vegetable or side green salad with your dish instead—and dressing on the side.

- ▶ **Dress your pizza perfectly.** Go for a plain and simple pizza with fresh vegetables, instead of meat. If whole-wheat crust is available, make that your choice.

No matter what kind of restaurant you're going to, there are certain things to keep in mind that will help you stay on course. Follow these tips and you'll be a healthy dining-out expert in no time. When you eat any dinner out, the salt content will be higher than what you are used to. That's why I remind readers to avoid weighing for at least 3 days after their Super Splurge—you need to allow your body to get rid of the excess water via urine.

Furthermore, don't skip your breakfast and skinny lunch during the day, thinking it'll help you save room for your restaurant meal.

You'll only end up overeating. Instead, eat regular meals from the Fat Blaster Meal Plan. If you're worried about self-control in a restaurant setting, try filling up on cut-up veggies or an apple and water before you head out for the night.

Don't be shy about asking for what you want the way you want it. If you see something you like on the menu but it is fried or made with butter, politely ask for the item to be grilled or sautéed with olive oil instead. And if you want the dressing on the side of your salad, ask for it that way. Most restaurants will be happy to comply.

As soon as you're seated at the restaurant, order a broth-based soup or a salad. Both these options have a lot of water in them, which will fill you up without filling you out, so you'll eat less overall at your Super Splurge meal.

Here are a few of my favorite Super Splurge menus when I go out with family and friends. Let me know your favorites!

ITALIAN FOOD 1 piece of lasagna, 7-layer salad, 1 piece of garlic bread, ½ cup of frozen yogurt (no topping, or forgo the bread and pick 1 topping)

PIZZA 2 medium-sized pieces of pizza with choice of meat and veggies, side salad, and 1 beer.

FAST FOOD 1 hamburger with veggie toppings; baked sweet potato fries or 1 small order of regular fries; side salad; ½ cup ice cream, 1 small cookie, or 1 brownie of choice; or 1 beer or glass of wine.

ASIAN CUISINE 2 orders of sushi, edamame, miso soup, salad with sliced avocado with grilled salmon, 1 glass of sake. If you don't want the salad, you can increase the sushi order to 3.

THAI FOOD 1 split order of a Thai main course entree, papaya and shrimp salad, 1 split order of Pad Thai, 1 order of mango and sticky rice or coconut ice cream.

MEXICAN FOOD 10 chips with salsa, 2 soft corn tortillas (shrimp, chicken, or beef) or bean tacos with side of guacamole, side of beans or rice (not both), or substitute fajitas for tacos and eat with 2 soft corn tortillas, 1 margarita.

AMERICAN CUISINE 1 side salad; filet of beef, strip steak, or ribs; baked potato with 1 tablespoon of sour cream; order of broccoli or other vegetable.

 PICK THE SMART SIDE

When eating out, always go for the baked potato or rice instead of French fries, potatoes au gratin, or scalloped potatoes; steamed spinach instead of creamed; and steamed rather than fried or sauced veggies. You'll save hundreds of calories and, I promise, you'll never miss them!

CHAPTER 6

SKINNY STRATEGY #4: LOSE WEIGHT EVEN FASTER!

*Nothing sets you up for success better
than a great breakfast!*

—*Denise*

Do you always snack while watching TV? Maybe you meet friends at night for dessert or coffee? Some of my girlfriends admit to night-time eating, especially when they are bored or stressed. The problem is that nighttime eating can set you up for big weight gain. Not only do people tend to ingest higher-calorie foods and drinks for snacks at night, but the time is typically spent sitting or lying down while watching TV, playing video games, or working on the computer.

In this fourth strategy, I will show you a new "skinny" way to live, as you learn why it is important to stop eating between dinnertime and breakfast. With the 7-Day Fat-Blast Diet, I will ask you to close up the kitchen after dinner. I will explain the latest science on this, too.

EATING AT NIGHT

An interesting study conducted on mice and published in the prestigious journal *Obesity* shows that fasting between the dinner meal and breakfast can kick-start the metabolism and speed up weight loss. We know that not eating after the last meal of the day gives the body enough time to burn all of the stored glycogen, plus some fat at night.

In the study, the obese mice that binged day and night developed all sorts of health problems like high LDL cholesterol, high blood glucose, metabolic disease, and fatty liver disease, which is an increasingly common problem among Americans. The mice that ate the same number of calories, but during a restricted time, had few signs of liver disease, high LDL cholesterol, or high blood sugar. As an amazing advantage, the mice that ate only during the restricted time had the greatest endurance of all the rodents in the study.

Ok, we're not mice! Still, this diet study gives us clues that our human body—the brain, stomach, and digestive system—needs some regular rules when it comes to managing the calories we ingest. This study suggests if we—like the obese mice—eat and eat anytime we want, the result may be metabolic collapse, with a fatty liver, high LDL cholesterol, spikes in blood sugar, and weight gain.

Staying up late and eating at night is a new experience and one that is difficult to break. When our grandparents went to bed with the chickens, they turned the lights off (or blew out the candles) and slept! But today with all the modern technology and power of the internet, we can connect with anyone 24 hours a day. There is no

 BREATHING CALMS YOU DOWN

I believe that breathing really helps to center you. Try to take deep breaths throughout the day. I do this every hour on the hour so I don't need a reminder to breathe deeply. Breathing properly gives you more energy and expands your lungs. Breathe in through your nose and breathe out from your abdomen. If your chest is rising, you are not breathing properly. I like to think about lengthening my body from the crown. Especially when you are under stress, take a few deep breaths to calm the body and lower the heart rate and blood pressure.

longer a cut-off time that is common among us—a time to shut down, relax, and stop eating.

Think of all the temptations you face each night—from mouth-watering commercials on TV whetting your appetite, to fast food restaurants just minutes away, to free delivery for just about any delectable concoction you might want. If you travel, there is the temptation of room service, late dinners with alcohol, or concessions just around the corner. The problem is, our metabolisms are sluggishly doing their best to digest the late night snacks when, in fact, many scientists theorize we are made to anticipate a fast at night—a time of restriction from eating, during which the body begins to burn fat.

With the 7-Day Fat-Blast Diet, I want you to eat most of your calories before 7 p.m. Let your last meal (dinner) be the end of your eating each evening. The reason is because your metabolism is the highest during the first 12 hours after waking. During this time, you burn a reported 75 percent of your daily caloric intake. That's a lot of calories to burn! If you "starve" all day like many people and eat the bulk of your calories at night—a late dinner with your spouse or colleagues, some dessert with your kids while watching TV, or a midnight snack—your body may not be metabolizing the calories as efficiently. So, here's my rule:

▶ Eat most of your calories between 7 a.m. and 7 p.m.

▶ Close down the kitchen from 7 p.m. to 7 a.m.

 ## TO AVOID STRESS EATING AT NIGHT, TREAT YOURSELF WELL

If you had an unusually stressful day or just finished a big, stressful project, go ahead and reward yourself! Not with food, of course, but with something that will help you relax. Instead, go get a pedicure or massage, take a long bubble bath, or read a good book.

WHAT ABOUT THE NIGHT SHIFT?

If you work the night shift, plan on fasting 12 hours after your last meal. For instance, if you wake up to go to work at 7 p.m., work until 7 a.m., and eat dinner at 8 a.m., go ahead and sleep. You can begin eating again at 8 p.m. If you work until midnight and eat at 1 a.m., then your first meal will be at 1 p.m. the next day. The idea of fasting after your last meal of the day can work with any schedule, just figure out the numbers. Once you understand the concept, make it work for you.

Ok, so now you understand the nighttime fast in Skinny Strategy #4. What do you do after not eating for 12 hours? You eat. You'll be hungry for breakfast as soon as you awaken, and this is a good thing! I love breakfast. Breakfast gives your body that all-important first oomph so you can make it through your day feeling fantastic. After a great night's sleep, I cannot wait to sip a mug of warm water or green tea with fresh lemon and a slice of ginger in it. First thing when I get up, I squeeze ½ of a fresh lemon in a mug of warm tap water, and then look forward to starting my day, feeling clean and renewed. I want you to do this, too!

YOUR EARLY MORNING OOMPH!

Breakfast is a great opportunity to get your day off to a healthy start. But did you know that eating a good breakfast could help rein in your appetite for the rest of the day? Breakfast jump-starts your metabolism, increases blood sugar, and boosts your energy so you "break the

 LAUGHTER IS GOOD MEDICINE

Humor is fabulous for your overall well-being. My husband Jeff makes me laugh every single day. But did you know that laughter also tones your tummy muscles? I love it. I tell my friends to laugh hard, laugh often, and enjoy the slimming results. Nothing funny going on? Pop your favorite comedy in the DVD player, or go online to see funny videos.

fast" and starting moving and thinking. Breakfast keeps you from snacking and binge-eating at lunch and dinner. Pretty great, right?

As you will see from the meal plans in this program, breakfast foods can be sweet or savory, depending on your preference. This morning meal can be very simple yet filling—a container of low-fat yogurt, some blueberries, a few walnuts for protein and good fats, and a cup of green tea. If you feel like eating a piece of leftover chicken breast, that works just fine, too.

Remember, breakfast should be easy to prepare most days, because I know you are busy. Some of my favorite breakfast foods include a slice of whole-grain toast with peanut butter and all-fruit jam, a white-corn omelet (page 204), or a bowl of oatmeal sprinkled with seasonal berries and cinnamon. Simple, nutrient-rich foods are really all it takes.

Bring Your Breakfast to Work Day

If you are strapped for time in the early morning hours, you can even bring your breakfast along to work with you. Take a plastic container

 LIVE IN THE MOMENT

Have you heard of being mindful? Mindfulness means paying attention to the present moment. Being aware of the actions you take and the choices you have control over—that is what will help you meet your goals and improve your life. For example, when you eat, don't just put food in your mouth or snack blindly because you are stressed or preoccupied. Pay attention to your portion sizes and think about whether you are already feeling full. Being mindful helps you enjoy your meals and keeps you on the path toward a healthy body weight. Are there any times at night when you find yourself snacking without thinking—in front of the TV, roaming through the refrigerator, after a stressful day? Make a point to pause, take a few deep breaths, and try to refocus on the here and now. You can do it!

filled with dry, ready-to-eat high-fiber cereal; a baggie of blueberries; and a 1-serving carton of skim milk. Now, that is the way to get healthier and skinnier.

7 Tips to Avoid Nighttime Hunger

To stay with Strategy #4 and avoid nighttime hunger, here are my 7 best tips:

1. **Clear out your cabinets and refrigerator** (page 28). If you don't have tempting snack foods sitting in your pantry, you can't indulge. Even if a snack seems to be "good for you"—you may want to keep it out of the pantry your first 5 weeks on the diet. Even healthy foods can result in weight gain if you haven't included these foods in your calorie count each day. It will get better—and easier, I promise!

2. **Ask a family member or friend to keep you honest.** If you get hungry an hour after dinner, buddy up and ask someone to hold you accountable to the 7-Day Fat-Blast Diet. Maybe they will talk with you on the phone if they don't live with you. Or go for a walk with someone until the hunger subsides.

3. **Stick with the recommended menu plan for the 7-Day Fat-Blast Diet.** If you are skipping meals like breakfast or lunch, you will be hungry at night as your body tries to compensate for the missing calories.

4. **Slow down when you eat.** It takes time (about 20-to-30 minutes) for your brain to get the message from your stomach that you are full. Put your fork down every few bites to help slow you down. Chew your food well, and sip water or another calorie-free beverage.

5. **Drink water with your meals.** Stopping to sip water or another non-caloric beverage while you eat helps slow you down, keeps you hydrated, and fills you up! Remember, I recommend

8 8-ounce glasses of water daily for good health, so sipping water with dinner helps you to meet that quota.

6. **Start meals with a soup or a salad.** The water content (and the fiber in the vegetables) makes you feel more satisfied, so you'll eat less of the main course. I like to keep bagged salads from the supermarket in my refrigerator vegetable bin, so I always have a fresh salad to use at mealtime. Be sure to wash any bagged salad or vegetables to make sure they are clean prior to eating them.

7. **Sip flavorful herbal tea.** There are many varieties of decaffeinated herbal tea—blackberry, acai-mango, orange-tangerine, apple-cinnamon, lemon-ginger—that really calm hunger pangs and leave you feeling satisfied. You can get packages of herbal tea that contain several different types. You can drink herbal tea hot or iced. Add a squeeze of lemon, lime, or orange to give it more zest. Think of it as a no-calorie dessert that you can have anytime!

 THE BENEFITS OF YOGA

Yoga is an ancient philosophy involving the unity of mind, body, and spirit that originated in India. It incorporates an approach to achieving enlightenment through specific breathing exercises, meditation, and physical postures called asanas, also known as yoga poses. I practice yoga every night because the postures stretch and strengthen my muscles, improve circulation, and energize my entire body. Plus, they're incredibly relaxing, and take away all the tension of the day so I can sleep like a baby. Trust me, you'll be glad you added yoga, with all its benefits, to your workouts.

CHAPTER 7

SKINNY STRATEGY #5: TOP 14 *SIDE EFFECT: SKINNY* FOODS

The foods you're eating should work for you,
not against you!

—*Denise Austin*

In this fifth Skinny Strategy, I want to tell you about some powerful foods—I call them *Side Effect: Skinny* Foods—that actually resemble the organ or body site they help. These foods are important. As you eat *Side Effect: Skinny* Foods at meals or snack time, I want you to remember the visual link between the food and the organ or body site to reinforce the importance of including these in your daily diet.

Not only do the *Side Effect: Skinny* Foods help you lose weight, they also boost the functioning of various parts of your body such as your heart, brain, eyes, skin, and more. Special nutrients found

 MY SKINNY SMOOTHIE TIP

I make fruit smoothies for my family in a blender, using red grapes, frozen blueberries and strawberries, a fresh banana, a splash of apple or orange juice, a cup of Greek yogurt, and some ice cubes. The girls and I drink this in the summer on the way to play tennis.

in these 14 foods support your body's growth, repair, and wellness. The nutrients include vitamins, minerals, amino acids, essential fatty acids, and water, and the calorie sources of carbohydrate, protein, and fat.

1. Carrots Protect Your Eyes

Is your vision getting blurry as you age? Then eat more carrots if you'd like to see clearly the rest of your life. When you slice a large carrot, you can actually see that it looks like the human eye with a pupil, iris, and radiating lines. Now when you slice up carrots for a dinner salad or afternoon snack, I want you to mentally associate this vegetable with healthy vision! Here are some ways carrots help you:

▶ Carrots are full of the phytochemical carotenoids that have antioxidant properties, protecting your eyes from free radicals, unstable molecules that cause cellular damage. An overproduction of free radicals results in damage that leads to cataracts, macular degeneration, and glaucoma.

 CARROTS ARE EYE CANDY

Carrots are full of the phytochemical, lutein. A study in the *British Journal of Nutrition* reports that lutein reduces the chance of cataracts by up to 40 percent. Here are 7 other foods also high in lutein:

1. Carrots

2. Kale

3. Spinach

4. Beets

5. Collard greens

6. Sweet red peppers

7. Eggs (yolk)

- Antioxidants in carrots help improve immunity and reduce the risk of disease such as cancer and heart disease.

GET THE SKINNY ½ cup of carrots has 25 calories, 2 grams of fiber, and 224 percent of your daily value of vitamin A.

2. Tomatoes Boost a Healthy Heart

When I slice tomatoes for my family's dinner salad I know I'm doing something good to protect our hearts! In fact, just like the human

 ORGANIC OR NOT?

While there is currently no solid research that proves that organic foods are better for you, there *are* several good reasons to buy organic, and several things to keep in mind when you're buying organic:

- Organic foods are better for the environment. Produce that's labeled USDA Certified Organic is grown without the use of pesticides, synthetic fertilizers, or genetically modified organisms, and organic meats and dairy products are free of antibiotics and growth hormones. Organic food supports local farmers who use renewable resources and promote soil and water conservation.

- Because organic foods often cost more for farmers to produce and are more expensive at the supermarket, you may want to be selective about which organic foods you get.

- When it comes to produce, the fruits and vegetables that are most likely to contain pesticide residues are ones that you would rinse before eating such as peaches, apples, berries, bell peppers, and spinach. Non-organic foods that have heartier skins, like bananas, oranges, avocados, and sweet peas, are less likely to be contaminated.

But whether or not you go organic, the most important thing is that you make all your food choices healthy ones!

heart, tomatoes are bright red with 4 chambers. Here's how tomatoes help your heart:

▶ Tomatoes are jam-packed with the antioxidants vitamin C and lycopene.

▶ In one study, people with high blood pressure who ate just 2 servings of tomatoes daily saw a large drop in blood pressure.

GET THE SKINNY 1 tomato has 22 calories, 1.5 grams of fiber, and 1.1 grams of protein.

3. Red Grapes Increase Blood Flow

Ever think that grapes look a bit like blood cells, especially with the dark-red, bluish-purple color? The latest nutritional research shows that eating grapes may protect your circulatory system. Here's why:

▶ Filled with natural polyphenols, grapes lower high blood pressure, boost blood flow, and reduce inflammation—all of which reduce your risk of heart disease and stroke.

▶ Grapes are power-packed with the phytochemical ellagic acid that has been found to prevent cancer.

 TOP 7 SUPER ANTIOXIDANT FOODS

1. Small red beans

2. Blueberries

3. Red kidney beans

4. Pinto beans

5. Cranberries

6. Artichokes

7. Blackberries

► An antioxidant called activin has been discovered inside the seeds of red grapes. Studies show that activin is up to 7 times more powerful as an antioxidant than vitamins C, E, and beta-carotene. By-products of the red grape, including wine, juice, or seeds, may offer significant protection against some types of cancer, heart disease, and other chronic illness.

GET THE SKINNY 1 cup of red or green grapes has about 100 calories, 1 gram of fiber, and 1 gram of protein.

4. Walnuts Make Bigger Brains

Sometimes walnuts remind me of a miniature brain with the two hemispheres, the cerebrums, and cerebellums. Is it any wonder walnuts are nicknamed "brain food?" Here's why walnuts boost bigger brains:

► Walnuts boost the growth of new, healthy, brain cells, which is important to anyone of any age.

► Filled with protein and super healthy fats such as omega-3 fatty acids, walnuts help decrease inflammation, boost immunity, and prevent autoimmune diseases and Alzheimer's disease.

 SAY YES TO GOOD FAT

Add these best fats to your diet:

Monounsaturated fat is a good-for-you fat. You'll find it in avocados, nuts, peanut oil, canola oil, tahini, and olives.

Omega-3 fats are really important, too! These fats are found in fatty fish (anchovy, mackerel, salmon, sardines, shad, and tuna), flaxseed, and nuts.

Polyunsaturated fat lowers LDL cholesterol and comes from oils that are liquid or soft at room temperature such as corn, safflower, sesame, soy bean, and sunflower oils.

GET THE SKINNY 1 ounce of walnuts has about 170 calories, 2 grams of fiber, and 7 grams of protein. Nuts are a super source of magnesium, vitamin E, and omega-3 fatty acids.

5. Ginger Calms the Tummy and Revs the Metabolism

Have you ever sipped ginger ale or snacked on ginger snaps when your tummy was upset? I know I have. Ginger is a medicinal herb that has anti-nausea effects. In addition, I think ginger sort of resembles the human stomach. Also, the spicy component of ginger helps to rev up the metabolism! Here's why ginger is one of my favorite *Side Effect: Skinny* Foods:

▶ Ginger helps the body to break down protein and fat and convert the food you ingest into energy.

▶ Findings suggest that ginger has a wealth of healing properties including anti-inflammatory, anti-hypertensive, and glucose-sensitizing actions.

GET THE SKINNY 1 teaspoon of grated ginger (serving size) has 2 calories.

 SAY NO TO BAD FAT!

Avoid adding these fats to your diet:

Saturated fat comes from animal sources and is found in red meat, butter, cheeses, luncheon meats, cocoa butter, coconut oil, palm oil, and cream.

Hydrogenated fat can raise your LDL cholesterol and is made during a chemical process called hydrogenation.

Trans fats are formed when unsaturated vegetable oils are hydrogenated to make them solid at room temperature (stick margarine).

TOP 7 OMEGA-3 FOODS

1. Flaxseed oil, flaxseed

2. Fish oil

3. Chia seeds

4. Mackerel

5. Sunflower seeds

6. Salmon

7. Olive oil

6. Kidney Beans Help Maintain Kidney Function

Red kidney beans rank second highest in antioxidants among all beans, but they rank at the top for me! If you look at a kidney bean, it almost resembles the human kidneys. While these protein-packed beans are not relegated to just kidney health, they do provide nearly 60 percent of your daily folate needs and are high in manganese and vitamin K, both cell protectors that reduce the chances of cancer. Here's even more good news about kidney beans:

▶ 1 cup of cooked kidney beans gives you about half of your daily fiber requirement. Fiber is important for regulating blood glucose levels and for bowel regularity.

▶ Kidney beans are high in magnesium, the "anti-stress mineral," which is vital for a healthy heart.

GET THE SKINNY ½ cup of red kidney beans has 125 calories, 6 grams of fiber, and 7 grams of protein. Women who might get pregnant should get 400 micrograms (mcg) of folic acid each day to reduce the chances of birth defects in the brain and spine of newborns.

7. Bok Choy Builds Stronger Bones

Bok choy, a nutritious cruciferous vegetable that looks similar to your bones, is a good source of calcium. Too little calcium intake can lead to osteoporosis or weak, brittle bones that fracture easily. Calcium is also vital in preventing high blood pressure and easing PMS symptoms. While the calcium content of bok choy does not compare to dairy products, it is a viable source of calcium for vegans or those who need to avoid dairy.

▶ Bok choy is full of indoles, special cancer-preventing enzymes that make estrogen less active.

▶ Rich in potassium, a mineral necessary for healthy nerve and muscle functioning, bok choy is also high in vitamin A, which is important for beautiful skin and eyes.

GET THE SKINNY 1 cup of shredded bok choy has 20 calories, 2 grams of fiber, and 3 grams of protein.

 TOP 7 VEGETABLES WITH INDOLES

1. Bok choy

2. Broccoli

3. Cabbage

4. Brussels sprouts

5. Collards

6. Turnip greens

7. Kale

8. Avocados Improve Uterine Health

Not only are avocados the same oval shape as a uterus, they are high in folic acid, which has been found to be important for reproductive health. Here's more on how they will help you get super healthy!

► Avocados are powerhouses of monounsaturated fats, which reduce the chances of the precancerous condition, cervical dysplasia.

► In addition, they have the highest fiber content of any fruit at 10 grams per avocado, and are filled with magnesium, potassium, and vitamins C and E.

GET THE SKINNY 1 avocado has 227 calories, 9 grams of fiber and 3 grams of protein.

9. Sweet Potatoes Keep the Pancreas Healthy

Sweet potatoes look like the pancreas and actually balance the glycemic index. Here's how:

► The carotenoids in sweet potatoes can stabilize blood glucose because they help the body respond to insulin.

► Sweet potatoes have a high content of soluble fiber that helps to reduce blood glucose levels.

GET THE SKINNY 1 sweet potato has 105 calories, 4 grams of fiber, and 2 grams of protein.

 MY SKINNY DIET TIP

I like to serve baked potatoes as a base for a healthy dinner. We top them with vegetables, salsa, cheese, and a little light butter for a quick and easy meal.

TOP 10 ENERGY FOODS

Many women avoid diets because they complain of having no energy. The 7-Day Fat-Blast Diet is a high-energy diet, filled with nutritious, natural, energizing, and delicious complex carbohydrates! Foods that are wrapped in their natural packaging such as hulls or peels rather than stuck in boxes or bags are the best energy blasters you can eat. Boost the nutrition in your diet with these rev-you-up foods:

► Black beans (or any legume)

► Brown rice

► Greens (kale, Swiss chard, mustard, collard, spinach)

► Crayon-colored fruit (berries, oranges, tomatoes)

► Brilliant colored vegetables (eggplant, red/yellow/orange bell peppers, sweet potatoes

► Oatmeal (my favorite!)

► Popcorn (air-popped with a few spritzes of liquid butter)

► Potatoes, small to medium-sized, and naked rather than loaded (I love my Idaho potatoes!)

► Quinoa

► Whole wheat

10. Grapefruits Keep Breasts Healthy

Grapefruits resemble the mammary glands of the female and are powerhouses of vitamin C, which acts like an antioxidant. But did you know that grapefruits also contain flavonoids, including naringenin? In some studies, naringenin was found to decrease the growth and increase the self-destruction of cancerous tumors of the breast. Here's more:

► Naringenin reduces inflammation and boosts special enzymes that deactivate carcinogens.

- ▶ Grapefruit pulp contains D-glucarates, which are healing compounds that suppress inflammation and cell proliferation and may help in the prevention of breast cancer.

- ▶ Want smoother skin? Eat more grapefruit! Grapefruit boosts collagen in the body, which is essential to keep skin looking young.

GET THE SKINNY ½ grapefruit contains 52 calories, 2 grams of fiber, and 1 gram of protein.

11. Milk Boosts Healthy Bones and Teeth

Many experts tell people to avoid "white foods"—white sugar, white flour, and white bread. I believe the color white in milk and other dairy products is a natural reminder of the need to build strong bones and teeth with natural calcium, a mineral. Here's why milk is necessary for a healthy body and bones:

- ▶ Calcium may help in preventing and treating high blood pressure and easing symptoms of PMS.

- ▶ Not getting enough milk? A low calcium intake can lead to early osteoporosis, the brittle bone disease that results in painful fractures, even death.

 HOW MUCH CALCIUM IS ENOUGH?

Young children (1 to 3 years old)—500 mg

Children (4 to 8 years old)—800 mg

Adolescents and young adults (9 to 18 years old)—1,300

Adults (19 to 50 years old)—1,000 mg

Pregnant and nursing women—1,000 to 1,300 mg

Senior adults (50+ years old)—1,200 mg

GET THE SKINNY 1 cup of skim milk (non-fat) contains 86 calories and 8 grams of protein. Just 3 servings of dairy products daily can keep your bones strong.

12. Berries Protect Blood Vessels

Some berries are the same color as blood and have been shown to be helpful with protecting blood vessels in diabetics. Here's what the latest studies show:

▶ Findings presented at the American Chemical Society suggest that berries keep your brain healthy through the aging process and also fight harmful free radicals and reduce inflammation.

▶ In one study, people with high blood pressure who ate berries daily saw a 7-point dip in their systolic blood pressure (the top number) after just 8 weeks.

GET THE SKINNY 1 cup of blueberries contains 84 calories, 4 grams of fiber, and 1 gram of protein.

 TOP 7 SKINNY FOODS FOR GLOWING SKIN

1. Salmon to calm inflammation

2. Cantaloupe with lycopene for a healthy glow

3. Berries with polyphenols for anti-aging and to fight wrinkles

4. Olive oil to beat dryness and roughness

5. Greens (broccoli, spinach, collards, mustards, kale) with antioxidants to keep skin elastic and zinc to build collagen

6. Carrots with beta-carotene to discourage wrinkles

7. Oatmeal with cleansing compounds to oust toxins

The very top way to keep your skin hydrated and supple and defeat dryness is to drink plenty of water. I drink 64 ounces of water every day. You should too!

13. Almonds for Strong Nails

Almonds are at the top of my *Side Effect: Skinny* Foods list! Almonds play a key role in healthy skin, hair, and nails—and they look like perfectly shaped fingernails too.

▶ These nuts are powerhouses of essential fatty acids, especially omega-3 fatty acids.

GET THE SKINNY 1 ounce of almonds contains 170 calories, 3 grams of fiber, and 6 grams of protein.

14. Plums for Gorgeous Skin

There is nothing more smooth and shiny than a ripe plum! This perfect fruit reminds me of our skin, especially our rosy cheeks. What's interesting is plums are rich in nutrients that help the skin maintain moisture and even more health-boosting benefits:

▶ Plums are filled with potassium, iron, vitamin K, and vitamin C.

▶ Prunes (dried plums) are packed with fiber and contain the natural laxative sorbitol.

GET THE SKINNY 1 plum is 30 calories and has 1 gram of fiber.

 CALM DOWN WITH BANANAS

Bananas are filled with vitamin B6 and tryptophan—both important for promoting a sense of calmness when life's stressors cause you to feel tense. Vitamin B6 is important for the synthesis of serotonin and dopamine, neurotransmitters that are necessary for healthy nerve cell communication. Tryptophan is an amino acid that stimulates serotonin, the neurotransmitter that has a calming effect on the body.

3 More Bonus Foods!

Here are 3 more of my favorite foods that are low in calories and high in the ability to lower inflammation in the body. Not only does inflammation trigger pain, but also it increases the chance of chronic diseases.

1. Cherries

Cherries contain the compound cyanidin, which is thought to block pro-inflammatory chemicals in the body. Inflammation is an important trigger for chronic conditions such as type 2 diabetes, pain problems, and cancer.

2. Oranges

Oranges have the anti-inflammatory flavonoid nobiletin. Hesperidin, another flavonoid that may reduce inflammation, is found in the thin, orange portion of the citrus peel.

3. Pineapple

Pineapple is filled with bromelain, an enzyme that helps reduce inflammation and pain. This delicious fruit is filled with manganese, a bone-building mineral, and vitamin C, which help to strengthen collagen.

CHAPTER 8

SKINNY STRATEGY #6: DOUBLE-YOUR-METABOLISM FOODS

*Release yourself from the power you are giving
your mirror and those around you—take control of who
you are and how you feel!*

—Denise

You're probably thinking, what's the real "trick" to my 7-Day Fat-Blast Diet? After all, the menu plan is delicious and filling, plus you get a Super Splurge once a week to satisfy any sweet cravings. My exercises are easy to learn and fun! You can work the Interval Walking, 7-Minute Slimmers, and Do-It-Yourself Tummy Tucks into your daily routine and even invite family, friends, and colleagues to join you.

Now I'm excited to share with you a few "magic" foods—what I call Double-Your-Metabolism Foods—that you can include in your daily diet to get the upper edge (a real boost) and get skinnier and healthier quickly and safely. The bulk of the 7-Day Fat-Blast Diet is based on a variety of colorful fruits and vegetables and whole grains that are filled with phytochemicals (phytonutrients). These chemicals or nutrients are derived from plants and provide a beneficial effect on health, as well as play an active role in preventing disease. Not only are these foods filled with fiber that helps to prevent conditions such as type 2 diabetes, heart disease, and cancer, but fruits, vegetables, and whole grains are low in calories and fill you up—not out.

AN APPLE A DAY KEEPS THE MUFFIN TOP AWAY

Because apples are one of my favorite fill-me-up fruits, I was intrigued with a study from the University of Iowa, confirming that a substance known as ursolic acid in apple peel may help to reduce obesity and associated health problems by increasing the amount of muscle and brown fat, two tissues in the body that are recognized as fantastic calorie burners. While further studies are needed, researchers are hopeful that the ursolic acid in apple peel may help increase skeletal muscle, reduce obesity, and prevent pre-diabetes and fatty liver disease, which affects more than 1 in 5 Americans.

Apples are rich in a soluble fiber called pectin that helps fill you up so you don't snack between meals. Pectin prevents blood-sugar spikes that cause your body to store fat and keeps you from having blood-sugar crashes with out-of-control cravings. In addition, pectin lowers the amount of calories and sugar that goes into your bloodstream after you eat.

SPICE UP YOUR FAT BLAST

Do you love spicy salsa as much as I do? I generously spoon salsa on my family's omelets, steamed vegetables, and baked potatoes and love the healthy zing it adds to plain dishes.

But did you know that there is more to spicy salsa than meets the taste buds? Some findings show that salsa stimulates the metabolism from 15 to 20 percent. That is a fabulous boost, isn't it? The capsaicin that is found in cayenne, chili, and jalapeno peppers heats up the body and stimulates the metabolism to burn more calories.

How does it work? Research from Canada's Laval University reveals that eating hot peppers temporarily triggers the release of adrenaline and other stress hormones in your body. The stress hormones kick-start your metabolism to boost the rate of calorie burning. In addition, findings show that people who routinely eat peppers feel a lot fuller—a lot faster.

A study from the *Journal of Nutritional Science and Vitaminology* revealed that eating just 1 mere tablespoon of chopped green or red chilies boosts the body's production of heat and the activity of your sympathetic nervous system (SNS). This, in turn, causes the *fight or flight response*, which makes your heart speed up, your breathing quicken, and your face flush. The skinny result? A temporary metabolism spike of around 23 percent!

Also, the Asian spice turmeric used in curry dishes is filled with curcumin, the active ingredient. Some studies suggest that curcumin may control the metabolism of fats, which plays a major role in the development of obesity.

SIP THE POUNDS AWAY WITH GREEN TEA

Numerous studies advocate sipping green tea for weight loss. Green tea is filled with catechins, a phytochemical that appears to briefly increase thermogenesis (the rate at which calories are burned) and raises the metabolic rate. Some findings shows that drinking 2 to 4 cups of green tea daily may push the body to burn 17 percent more calories than normal over a short time period.

GREEN COFFEE EXTRACT SHOWS PROMISE

Green coffee bean extract is getting lots of buzz these days. While the jury is still out on green coffee bean extract, this natural supplement, which contains high concentrations of chlorogenic acids that are known to have health benefits, does appear to have some promise for short-term weight loss.

In a limited study published in the journal *Diabetes, Metabolic Syndrome and Obesity: Targets and Therapy*, researchers reported that 16 overweight adults lost an average of 17.5 pounds and 16 percent in body fat over a 22-week period while taking green coffee bean extract.

This same study, also presented at the American Chemical Society's meeting, revealed that participants who took the green coffee bean extract in supplement form reduced their body weight by 10.5 percent—all within 22 weeks and without changing their normal diet. In fact, the participants' intake of calories, carbs, fats, and protein did not change during the time of the study. Also, their exercise habits remained the same. Sound too good to be true?

It's thought that green coffee bean extract works by reducing the absorption of fat and glucose in the gut and maybe by reducing insulin levels. Watch for more confirmation studies to be announced or ask your doctor or nutritionist if this is safe for you to take.

CALCIUM REVS UP YOUR METABOLISM

Load up on dairy (low-fat, of course). Findings in the *American Society for Nutritional Sciences Journal of Nutrition* concluded that women who consumed milk, cheese, and yogurt 3 to 4 times a day lost 70 percent more body fat than women who didn't consume dairy.

It's believed that the calcium in dairy products revs up the metabolism. The best fat-blast appears to come from dairy products instead of foods fortified with calcium, like orange juice.

STAY FULLER, LONGER (NO KIDDING)

Along with some unique foods that rev up your metabolism, I also want you to add some "fill 'er up foods" that will help you to manage your ravenous appetite and prevent binge-eating. Here's what you must know!

BEFORE MY CAMERA SHOOT

Women ask me repeatedly, "What do you do before a camera shoot to look lean and trim?" I tell them the truth: I get lean, green, and clean! You don't have to be in front of the TV camera to want a lean, trim body. Because any picture (family photo or on TV) makes you look 10 pounds heavier, I always bring down the salt content of my meals. For 7 days before a photo shoot, I read labels, avoid soups and other canned foods, and eat minimal salt. Also, I don't use sugar in my coffee and eliminate any type of sugary foods that give me nothing but empty calories—this means no Super Splurge on the week before my camera shoot. I eat good carbs, such as oatmeal, 7 days before a shoot. And I thrive on hard-boiled eggs, tuna, and salmon to get plenty of EPA from omega-3 fatty acids to give me energy. I keep drinking 64 ounces of water a day and try to keep my urine clear, which means I'm getting ample water. Just like I recommend to you, I stay with my 7 a.m. to 7 p.m. eating rule to make sure all the food I eat is well metabolized.

Fiber is a Fat Fighter

Do you know that studies show if people ate the same diet—same calories, similar foods—except one diet is high in fiber and the other is low in fiber, those on the high-fiber diet will lose more weight? That is because fiber is a fat fighter!

Findings also show that thinner people eat more fiber than heavier people. Here are some ways fiber can help get rid of pounds and help you feel fuller, too:

FIBER IS A NATURAL APPETITE SUPPRESSANT. Foods high in fiber stop your blood sugar from spiking and allow your body to slowly digest the food. The result? You are not hungry, you eat less food, and you lose weight fast.

FIBER BLASTS FAT. Fiber removes as much as 5 percent of the fat in the foods you eat and carries waste out of your body quickly, taking unabsorbed fat and calories with it.

FIBER LOWERS INSULIN LEVELS. A high-fiber diet lowers blood sugar, which lowers insulin levels, and your body switches into the much-desired fat-burning mode.

To include more fiber in your diet, consider the following 7 tips:

1. Add beans to your dishes, specifically red, black, pinto, and great northern beans.

2. Munch on raw veggies, such as carrots and broccoli.

3. Look for high fiber cereals, meaning more than 3 grams of fiber per serving. Toss some raisins or other dried fruit or a diced apple in with your oatmeal.

4. Eat the whole fruit or vegetable, skins included, to maximize your fiber intake. And remember not to cook vegetables until they've lost their crunch. Opt for oatmeal or bran cereals for breakfast instead of crispy corn or rice.

5. Eat 100 percent whole-wheat bread for added fiber.

The American Dietetic Association recommends 25 to 35 grams of dietary fiber per day, which can help you to feel full and keep your blood-sugar levels normal.

Whole Grains Boost Weight Loss

For years, the top diets have all but banned whole grains, thinking that these carbohydrates would cause a sudden spike and subsequent drop in blood sugar, and result in increased hunger and weight gain. Now we know differently! Whole grains help keep blood glucose levels even, which can help lower the chance of metabolic syndrome and problems related to obesity.

Some findings show that it is the intake of refined grains, as opposed to whole grains, that is associated with weight gain and body fat distribution.

Whole-grain foods, including some breakfast cereals, barley, bran, brown rice, bulgur, and oatmeal, are high in water content and fiber. This added water and fiber can help protect against weight gain by making you feel full longer and therefore less likely to overindulge later on too many snacks.

Whole grains include all 3 parts of the grain kernel—the bran, germ, and endosperm—and are excellent sources of vitamins and minerals such as thiamin, riboflavin, niacin, vitamin E, magnesium, phosphorus, selenium, zinc, and iron. One fiber-packed serving of whole grains is equivalent to one of the following:

► 1 slice of sprouted wheat bread

► ½ cup of cooked brown rice

► 2 ounces of cooked oatmeal

► ½ cup of dry whole-grain cereal

► ½ cup of cooked whole-grain pasta

Unlike many weight-loss plans, the 7-Day Fat-Blast Diet urges you to include at least 2 servings of whole grains during the Level 2, and more once you enter the Forever Skinny (lifetime) level, selecting foods whose first ingredient contains the word *whole* instead of *enriched*.

Whole grains need twice as much water or liquid as regular grains (except for quick-cooking brown rice), and do not cook instantly. You can soak the grain overnight to reduce the cooking time. This works well with oats or brown rice.

Grapefruit Dissolves Fat

Some exciting new studies conclude that grapefruit is a healthy diet food that helps to dissolve fat and cholesterol. Grapefruits have more than 15 grams of pectin, a fat-blasting insoluble fiber that helps curb your appetite by expanding in your stomach. This helps you to feel full!

Also, grapefruit is packed with galacturonic acid, which gives this fruit its ability to blast the fat and cholesterol. Some nutritionists recommend eating ½ a grapefruit with each meal to help increase a feeling of fullness and weight reduction. I have included grapefruit on some of the 7-Day Fat-Blast Diet's menus!

Legumes Prevent Overeating

I eat tons of legumes! Beans, lentils, and peas are low in calories and are a "go to" food for many vegetarians. They are packed with carbohydrates, protein, and that much-needed fiber, and because they are slow to be digested, they help you feel full longer and keep you from overeating. Legumes help me move more and eat less!

Some new studies reveal that legumes contain the digestive hormone cholecystokinin (CCK), an appetite suppressant. In one study, research revealed that men who ate beans had double the cholecystokinin levels as those who ate a low-fiber diet. (I'm sure this works for women, too!)

Anthocyanins, a class of compounds found in dark red fruit like berries, are quite abundant in legumes. In black beans alone, the levels of anthocyanins are 10 times greater than all of the antioxidants found in oranges. Anthocyanins have been found to have the strongest anti-inflammatory effect of any flavonoid tested.

Pine Nuts Suppress Your Appetite

Nuts and seeds are a great source of omega-3 fatty acids, vitamin E, and magnesium. Some recent studies show that tiny pine nuts, the creamy seeds from pine trees, have the fatty acid that releases the appetite-suppressing hormone cholecystokinin (CCK) that sends signals of satiation to the brain, which diminishes the desire to eat.

In one particular study, women who ate pine nuts reportedly had less desire to eat only 30 minutes after ingesting the nuts. The pine nuts boosted appetite suppressors up to 60 percent for 4 hours! If this is proven with further studies, imagine snacking on some pine nuts before dinner and then feeling full after eating just half of your meal. Now that is how fat-blasting works!

The only drawback to nuts and seeds is the calorie count—it is relatively high. For example, 1 ounce of peanuts is about 165 calories, while 1 ounce of pine nuts is 190 calories. While I encourage you to include nuts and seeds like pine nuts, walnuts, and peanuts in your diet, it is also important to keep track of the serving size, as I have done in the suggested menus starting on page 144.

Protein Helps Control Hunger

The diverse protein choices on the 7-Day Fat-Blast Diet will keep you full and satisfied on my program. In Level 1, you will eat more protein-rich foods like eggs and fish and limit your complex carbohydrates to help control hunger and cravings, which will get you started

 7 PLANT SOURCES OF OMEGA-3 FATTY ACIDS

1. Walnuts

2. Tofu

3. Soybean products

4. Flaxseed

5. Flaxseed oil

6. Canola oil

7. Wheat germ

losing a lot of weight. Then after 3 weeks at this level, you will add more complex carbohydrates (low-starch vegetables, super-antioxidant fruits, and whole grains) to give you a steady weight loss as long as you need it.

As an example, breakfast most mornings on the first level of the 7-Day Fat-Blast Diet may be some type of egg recipe, using whole eggs, egg whites, and egg substitutes. Eggs are loaded with an essential amino acid called lutein, which provides a weight-loss advantage during dieting by helping to reduce loss of lean tissue, promote loss of body fat, and stabilize blood glucose levels. Eggs help to maintain lean muscle mass, which is crucial for long-term weight loss (muscle burns fat and calories).

Fish is another low-calorie, high-protein mainstay of this diet plan. Some fish, such as salmon, tuna, and trout, are filled with omega-3 fatty acids. Marine omega-3 fatty acids contain eicosapentaenoic acid (EPA) and docosahexaenoic acid (DHA), which are known to decrease inflammation in the body.

Here are some other powerful foods and ideas for how to eat them. I think you'll love these as much as I do!

ROASTED VEGETABLES Roasting vegetables is an easy way to bring out their unique flavors. Roasting slowly caramelizes the sugars and enhances the taste of any vegetable, even ones you think you may not like! Start with a solid, stainless steel baking sheet with edges. Use a small amount of extra-virgin, cold-pressed olive oil, fresh pressed garlic, and kosher salt. Make sure to pat dry your veggies before rubbing with oil. If your oven has a delayed cooking feature, you can prepare the veggies, put them in the oven before work, and have them ready to eat when you walk in the door. Simple, delicious, and healthy!

CHIA SEEDS Chia seeds are seeds from the salvia hispanica plant and are loaded with omega-3 fatty acids and fiber. Many people mistakenly believe chia seeds aid weight loss but recent studies have not confirmed this. Nevertheless, chia seeds are a great addition to any diet since they are super high in antioxidant, disease-fighting compounds.

GROUND FLAXSEED Like chia, flaxseed is very high in omega-3 fatty acids and fiber, both soluble and insoluble kinds. Ground flaxseed meal is a great way to add fiber to yogurts, cereals, and baked goods. Store covered in the refrigerator. Choose ground flax seeds over whole seeds and oil.

GREEN TEA Green tea has been cultivated for centuries. Of the 3 kinds of teas, oolong, black, and green, green tea contains the highest amount of polyphenols or antioxidants. These powerful plant chemicals may reduce the risk of developing heart disease and certain cancers. Green tea contains both caffeine and catechins making it a perfect mid-morning or afternoon pick me up. Catechins may be responsible for the tea's fat-burning effect.

KALE AND CHARD These super-charged greens are full of antioxidants and high in vitamin A. I love them crispy from the oven or as an addition to a smoothie. Hardy and tough, these can be grown in the garden, window box, or pot until frost.

LEMON This vitamin C–rich fruit brings out the flavors in all foods. I love to use it in dressings and as a final splash before serving veggies from the oven. Lemon zest (the yellow part of the peel), adds spice to not only vegetables, but fruits, as well.

MY FAVORITE SEASONINGS Forget the salt! Pressed garlic tops my favorite seasoning list. Use on baked fish and chicken, and on any kind of vegetable. Red pepper flakes add a kick to any dish, especially pasta, bean bowls, and soups. A spritz of orange juice adds just the right touch of sweetness to fruit and veggies. Fresh or dried cilantro, parsley, and basil all add fragrance and flavor. Keep these on hand to freshen up any dish.

MUSTARDS There are so many types of mustards, from tangy to pungent. I buy many kinds and have them on hand for dipping.

One of my favorite snacks is sliced turkey breast rolled up with an asparagus spear, roasted red pepper, and avocado and dipped a one of my special gourmet (not expensive) mustards.

CHOCOLATE I love chocolate, especially when trying to lose weight. That may seem contradictory, but chocolate increases well-being and adds just the right amount of satiation that many diets lack. So let yourself indulge in a few chocolate chips or a few squares of dark chocolate. Pair with fresh fruit or a handful of nuts to make it last longer.

PROTEIN Protein is so important for muscle growth and tissue repair. In this diet plan, proteins can be interchanged with one another. If the menu calls for fish but you prefer chicken or tur-key, choose what you like. Fish, chicken, turkey, and tofu can all be interchanged, but I recommend keeping red meat to no more than twice a week. I top proteins with pressed garlic before grilling or broiling.

EDAMAME Green soy beans in the pod make a perfect snack, espe-cially when you are looking for more than a few bites. Steam, boil, or microwave beans. Let cool and sprinkle with teriyaki sauce, pressed garlic, and lemon juice. Keep in the refrigerator for a ready-to-go, anytime snack.

EGGS In my menus, you will find many egg dishes for breakfast. I like egg whites because they are high in protein and low in calories, but you can throw a yolk in here and there.

NUTS AND SEEDS Nuts and seeds are full of healthy fats and fiber and are one of the quickest ways to keep hunger away. Contrary to popular belief, if you eat nuts instead of junk food, you will not gain weight. Of course you have to watch the serving size, but even a few nuts curb hunger fast. Add nuts and seeds to stir fry, sal-ads, cereals, and yogurt. Nut butters go well with apples, pears, and celery. A small handful in the afternoon can help you make it until dinner without stopping by the candy jar at work! They are a great pick-me-up before a workout. You can roast raw nuts over medium/low heat in a frying pan sans oil and add your favorite seasoning: cumin, garlic powder, low-sodium soy sauce, cayenne pepper, cinnamon, or cocoa for flavor. These spices and seasonings give nuts a kick and add pizzazz to an otherwise ho-hum afternoon.

CHAPTER 9

SKINNY STRATEGY #7: DAILY BODY BLITZ

*Beauty is feeling good about yourself, and
you can't buy it; you have to earn it!*

—*Denise*

How would you describe yourself: twitchy or calm? Restless or relaxed? Do you squirm while waiting in the long grocery line or rush-hour traffic? Maybe you pace back and forth while you think, or tap your fingers rhythmically on your computer desk while working.

If you are a natural-born fidgeter, you may have elevated non-exercise activity thermogenesis or NEAT. If you don't fidget, it may be part of why you're struggling with your weight.

Non-exercise activity thermogenesis (NEAT) is the energy used for everything you do that does not include eating, sleeping, or athletics. NEAT includes the energy you use while typing, walking to work, gardening, or even fidgeting. Researchers at Mayo Clinic have found that even small physical activities boost metabolism considerably and the cumulative effect of many actions each day result in a person's daily NEAT.

Some amazing research published in the journal *The Scientist* shows that people who are overweight tend to sit for about 150 minutes per day more than thin people.

This detailed study found that overweight people were far less fidgety than skinny people. They moved less. They did not fidget or pace. In fact, researchers revealed that overweight people spend around 2 hours a day simply sitting still.

According to the findings, lean people do the exact opposite: they pace, fidget, squirm, and move enough each day to burn about 350 additional calories. This is the equivalent to 10 to 30 pounds a year!

As you will learn in this last Skinny Strategy, the most effective way to lose weight and keep it off is to keep your body active—daily—moving every chance you get and keeping your cardiovascular system in optimal health. With this strategy, I will help you redefine everyday exercise to include tapping, stretching, fidgeting,

 ### 7 WAYS TO LOOK 7 POUNDS SLIMMER— TODAY!

Did you know that good posture can make you look 7 pounds slimmer? It really can! I want you to think about lengthening your body with good body alignment and great posture. Practice the following 7 steps every morning until they become natural for you:

1. Lift your upper body up off your hips to add an inch to your height.

2. Draw in your abs so your legs move more fluidly and gracefully.

3. Pull your shoulders down and back.

4. Slightly lift your chest bone (sternum).

5. Breathe deeply and let the oxygen flow into your back to keep your back muscles elastic.

6. Always pull in your core and abdominals, as you stand tall.

7. Look straight ahead and feel like your hair is in a high ponytail being pulled upwards. This visualization trick helps to elongate the neck.

pacing, shaking, and other enjoyable activities you can do any time of the day or night—even at work. When you combine the 7-Day Fat-Blast Diet and Workout with the Daily Body Blitz—another 20 minutes of physical activity—you will boost weight loss and good health!

NOW GET UP AND GET RESTLESS!

Turn idle time into toning time. Start pacing. Get up and dance—whatever you like! And in doing so, I guarantee you'll see the scale budge, and you'll lose weight even faster.

I love to do 1-minute Body Blitzes anytime throughout the day. You can do 5 in the morning, 5 at lunch, 5 in the afternoon, and then 5 before bedtime. That is an *added 20 minutes a day* of fat-burning exercise that will help you get healthier and skinnier even faster! Here's the rule I want you to follow: Whenever you find yourself waiting—sitting in an airplane, car, or train; seated at the doctor's office; watching your child play sports—find a way to move, even if all you do is tap your feet!

For instance, when I'm waiting for a flight at the airport, I try to walk the concourse instead of sitting at the gate. Whenever I'm in a grocery line, I do isometrics, tightening up various muscles in my body—my arms, my legs, my buns, my abs. I do each set for 5 seconds and then release. While brushing my teeth, I pace or do calf raises. I always check my posture, making sure my abs are zipped up as if I were trying to fit into a pair of tight jeans, and my shoulder blades are down, squeezed together and low on my back.

Periodically when working at home, I take short stretching and strengthening breaks. I place my palms on the kitchen counter, step back with my feet and bring my body into a right angle, reaching back with my tailbone as I scoop my abs up and in (like a modified *downward dog* in yoga).

Every hour, I do my Do-It-Yourself Tummy Tuck, as discussed on page 52. This simple exercise works wonders to flatten your belly and to make you look slim and trim!

EXERCISE ANYWHERE, ANYTIME

Muscles don't know if you're in a fancy gym or in your kitchen. These tips are designed for busy lives—a minute here and a minute there adds up. These are great ways to sneak in certain exercises throughout the day. Keeping your muscles toned works miracles for your metabolism

▶ To get a firm bottom when you're walking up stairs, always skip a step—you'll feel it more in your rear end. Always remember to squeeze your bottom.

▶ Keep a pair of 3-lb or 5-lb dumbbells at your desk and do lifts while you're talking on the phone, in-between meetings, and so on.

▶ In your car, do tummy tightners—pull in your stomach muscles and tighten for 5 seconds. It's equivalent to 1 sit-up.

▶ Do squats while you blow-dry your hair in the bathroom.

▶ Do leg lifts in the kitchen.

▶ Hula hoop for your waist line—it helps get circulation going and works the muscles of the entire torso. Play loud music and have fun with it.

▶ Use resistance bands for your arm workouts.

▶ Sit on a balance ball at your desk—it helps engage your ab muscles. Then you can roll the ball back and do a few sit-ups at the office, too.

MY TOP 20 BODY BLITZES

Think about all of the sitting you do: at your desk, in your car, in front of the TV with the remote control, at your computer, and on the weekends. Health experts warn us that spending an excessive amount of time sitting (more than 3 hours each day) shortens your life expectancy by 2 years when compared to people who spend less than 3 hours sitting each day. Some scientists put a sedentary lifestyle in the same risky arena as obesity and cigarette smoking when it comes to your health and longevity.

We've engineered inactivity into our lives. However, even if you are not a fidgeter, there are ways you can certainly act like one. It is not as hard as you might think.

Did you know you can burn up to 500 calories per day just by fidgeting? That is right! Just doing little exercises in your car, while you brush your teeth, while you are sitting at your computer, or while you read a book (like you are right now!) can burn calories, keep the oxygen flowing, and stretch and tone your muscles 1 minute at a time! These Body Blitzes take only 1 minute or less and they really do work! They don't replace your Interval Walking or 7-Minute Slimmers (Skinny Strategy #2), but you can use these moves to get in some extra fitness all day long!

1. MOVE AROUND YOUR OFFICE OR WORKSPACE AS OFTEN AS YOU CAN. Walk around, particularly if you are not a fidgeter. Although you may not be genetically predisposed to fidget, you can certainly learn the behavior over time.

2. WANDER AROUND WHEN YOU TALK ON YOUR CELL PHONE OR DURING AN OFFICE CONFERENCE CALL. You are getting the job done while burning more calories!

3. JOG IN PLACE WHILE WAITING FOR A BUS OR TRAIN. Be sure to hold in your abs too!

4. PICK THE PARKING SPOT FARTHEST AWAY FROM THE STORE. Not only will you save yourself the time of driving around trying to snag the closest spot you can find, but you'll burn off extra calories walking from your car to the store and back again.

5. TAKE RECESS AFTER LUNCH. You probably loved both recess and lunch when you were in school, so why not enjoy both again by taking a walk after lunch and getting some fresh air and exercise.

6. STAND UP AND STRETCH. If you're a commuter, give up your seat to someone else and spend the ride standing, or better yet, walking around and getting in a good stretch. Spending the commute standing, stretching, or walking will help relieve some of that stiffness from being parked at your desk all day.

7. GET UP AT THE OFFICE. Rather than emailing or phoning a colleague, make the trip to her office. And spread out your office errands, like copying or dropping something in the mail slot, so that you have to get up and move as many times as possible during the day.

8. CLIMB 2 FLIGHTS OF STAIRS. You burn up to 1 calorie per step. It adds up after a while!

9. GET UP AT HOME. Walk around during TV commercials. Ditch the remote control and change the channels manually. This forces you to move around more.

10. POWER WALK FOR 1 MINUTE. You can do this at home, at the office, around the block, at the mall.

11. DO A DIY TUMMY TUCK. Tighten your tummy muscles, release, and tighten them again.

12. BICYCLE AT YOUR DESK! Bicycle your legs as you sit at your desk. Go fast—up, down, up, down. Think of how many calories you are burning with each bicycle pump—and you're toning your tummy, too!

13. MARCH IN PLACE FOR 1 MINUTE. With your feet under your hips, march bringing your knees as high as possible. You can burn more calories by jogging in place for 1 minute!

14. REACH TO THE SKY. Stretch up with your hands and reach for the sky for 1 minute. Really reach high and feel your body stretch out.

15. DO PROGRESSIVE MUSCLE STRENGTHENING. Tighten muscles throughout your entire body for 1 minute, starting with your face and ending at your feet.

16. CRUNCH TIME! Get down on the floor and do 1 minute of crunches.

17. DO JUMPING JACKS. Do 1 minute of jumping jacks, starting with your feet under your hips and hands down by your side. Jump your feet out to the sides into a wide angle as you simultaneously lift your arms laterally out to the sides. Jump back in as you lower your arms.

18. WIPE IT DOWN. Wipe tabletops in your home or office; wipe a window or 2 and really move your body up and down as you do so.

19. DO AN ARABESQUE. Stand up nice and straight, lift 1 leg behind you, then bring it back down—this is just like an arabesque (back leg lift) in ballet. You can even do this while leaning over the sink and brushing your teeth.

20. STEP IT UP. Stand at the base of the stairs. Put your right foot on the step, and then place your left foot next to it. Now put your right foot back on the floor, and place your left foot next to it. Do this step up and step down for 1 minute to boost your heart rate.

JUST KEEP ON MOVING!

You need to know that for weight loss and better health, moving is far better than sitting around. Constantly think about where and when in your life you can burn a few more calories, because over time, it all adds up. It is worth the effort. Keep on moving for better health and a better figure!

CHAPTER 10

THE 7-DAY FAT-BLAST DIET AND WORKOUT: LEVEL 1

You hold the key to your weight-loss success.
It's all about your attitude!

—*Denise*

Before you begin Day 1 of the 7-Day Fat-Blast Diet and Workout, I want you to start your morning feeling fresh, clean, and natural! Here's what I do, and you can do it also every single morning—without fail.

1. **Sip a mug of warm water or your favorite herbal or green tea with ½ of a fresh squeezed lemon and a slice of fresh ginger in it.** I have found that this natural drink helps to regulate your body without harsh chemicals or calories. Ginger is soothing to your tummy, while lemons have diuretic properties and help flush fluids out of the body.

2. **Eat a few leaves of parsley.** My grandmother did this her entire life, and I follow her practice. Parsley contains health-boosting flavonoids that act as antioxidants and is a source of vitamins A, B (folic acid), and C. You can grow parsley in your garden or in an herb container on your windowsill.

LEVEL 1

Length of time: 3 weeks

GETTING STARTED Kick-start your metabolism and boost quick weight loss with a 21-day diet based on Calorie Confusion and a workout based on Muscle Confusion. You will change your calorie intake every 2 days as explained on page 167, and do the suggested exercises in Skinny Strategy #2. Do this diet and workout plan for 21 days before moving to Level 2. You won't see processed foods like mac and cheese on this 3-week jumpstart. Instead, I have based the menu on the very best whole foods that are far better for you than any processed box mix.

 CALORIE ALERT!

If you find this diet is too restrictive and you need more food or want to be closer to a 1400-calorie range, choose foods from the food group lists to make up the calorie difference from the menu you are eating that day. You can find these lists on page 208. Here are some tips to help you:

▸ Adding 1 carbohydrate serving will raise your calorie intake by approximately 100 calories.

▸ Adding 1 fat will raise your calorie intake by approximately 45 calories.

▸ Adding 1 protein serving (3 oz.) will raise your calorie intake by approximately 150 calories.

▸ Adding 1 fruit serving will raise your calorie intake by approximately 60 calories.

You can see it does not take much to up the calories! If you decide to add more options, choose wisely because a few extra calories can slow down your weight loss.

Now don't worry about counting calories. I have done the homework for you with calorie-controlled menus. If you follow each day's menu carefully, you won't have to count anything except all the pounds you lose.

The main goal of this book is to get healthy, but the bonus side effect is that you also get slim and fit. Interestingly, research speculates that a lower caloric intake may be the Fountain of Youth and help slow the aging process, increase brain function and longevity, and prevent heart disease, diabetes, and cancer. It is your job to put the diet into practice to get the super health benefits.

Another important rule: you need to eat your dinner meal by 7 p.m. to benefit from the plan. Studies find that people who stop eating at the dinner meal (meaning no snacking after your last meal of the day) and wait 12 hours before eating breakfast, lose weight much faster.

 ATTENTION VEGETARIANS AND VEGANS!

Be sure your diet is balanced. When you eliminate animal products, you have to make up for the important nutrients they contain such as vitamin B12, iron, and zinc. The U.S. Department of Agriculture has some great nutritional tips for vegans and vegetarians at *www.choosemyplate.gov*. Simply modify the suggested meals in the 7-Day Fat-Blast Diet with the appropriate substitutions to get the vitamins and minerals you need.

The 7-Day Fat-Blast Diet and Workout: **Level 1**
21-Day Jumpstart Plan

DAY 1

CALORIES: 1090

WORKOUT: STRETCHES AND INTERVAL WALKING

Breakfast

White Corn Scramble
Sliced tomatoes
1 slice turkey bacon
½ grapefruit

Fat-Blast Snack

20 grapes
⅛ cup chopped raw walnuts

Lunch

Fat-Blast Garden Mix
Add:
2 T. kidney beans
4 oz. of grilled chicken
1 T. Olive O Dressing

Fat-Blast Snack

½ cup carrot sticks, ½ cup red pepper strips, ½ cup cucumber slices
dipped in ¼ cup non-fat cottage cheese mixed with chives, pressed
garlic, and fresh chopped basil

Dinner

1 tomato, sliced; 1 oz fresh mozzarella; fresh basil; 2 T. diced red
onion
4 oz roasted chicken or turkey
Roasted vegetables: ¾ cup cauliflower, 1 bulb fennel, and ¾ cup
asparagus with pressed garlic

DAY 2

CALORIES: 1170

WORKOUT: STRETCHES AND 7-MINUTE SLIMMERS

Breakfast
Fat-Blast Fruit Energizer Smoothie (recipe on page 192)

Fat-Blast Snack
10 raw almonds
1 T. dried cherries

Lunch
Fat-Blast Asian Slaw (recipe on page 190)
Add:
1 T. dry roasted peanuts
½ cup shelled edamame
3 oz. shrimp, deveined, boiled
Roasted vegetables: 1 cup broccoli and ½ cup red pepper

Fat-Blast Snack
1 small container of yogurt (90 calories)
1 T. ground flaxseed

Dinner
Fat-Blast Garden Mix or 7-Layer Salad (recipe on page 200)
1 T. Olive O Dressing
4 oz lean beef, veggie, or turkey burger with 1 T. sautéed onions and
1 T. sautéed mushrooms (no bun)
1 slice of low-fat cheese
½ sliced tomato and 1 dill pickle spear
1 slice avocado

> **NOTE:** Substitute whole grains for any white flour products. The additional fiber will improve your health and keep you feeling full for a longer period of time.

DAY 3

CALORIES: 1270

WORKOUT: STRETCHES AND INTERVAL WALKING

Breakfast
2-egg-white spinach and feta cheese (2 T.) omelet
Salsa

Fat-Blast Snack
1 T. spicy pecans
Hot green tea

Lunch
3 oz. sliced turkey breast on 2 slices whole-wheat bread
Top with lots of fresh veggies
1 T. mustard
1 cup carrots, 1 bell pepper, with ⅓ cup hummus

Fat-Blast Snack
Tangerine

Dinner
Caesar salad with 1 T. choice of dressing
¾ cup pasta with tomato sauce and 2 T. Parmesan cheese
3 oz shrimp or scallops
1 cup sauté of onions and garlic
Crispy Kale

 1 MEAT SERVING EQUALS:

- ▸ 3 oz. meat, fish, or poultry
- ▸ 1–2 ounces sliced cheese
- ▸ ½ cup cottage cheese or ricotta
- ▸ 1 egg or 2 egg whites (or ¼ cup egg substitute)
- ▸ 2 tablespoons nut butter
- ▸ ½ cup beans

DAY 4

CALORIES: 1160

WORKOUT: STRETCHES AND INTERVAL WALKING

Breakfast

1 cup plain, low-fat yogurt
½ cup berries: sliced strawberries, raspberries, blueberries, black-berries (choose one or several types)
⅛ cup chopped raw walnuts

Fat-Blast Snack

Skinny latte or hot green tea

Lunch

Fat-Blast Garden Mix or 7-Layer Salad
Add:
½ oz roasted red peppers
2 oz grated low-fat cheese
4 oz sliced roast turkey or chicken breast

Fat-Blast Snack

4 stalks of celery
1 T. natural peanut butter

Dinner

1 cup Luscious Lentil Soup
Chicken lettuce wraps

 EAT GOOD FAT ON THE 7-DAY FAT-BLAST DIET

Be sure to choose unsaturated fats (found in fish, olives, nuts, seeds, oils, and avocados). Avoid saturated fat (found in animal products like butter, whole milk, and meat), as well as trans fat (found in margarine, shortening, and commercial baked goods).

DAY 5

CALORIES: 1100

WORKOUT: STRETCHES AND INTERVAL WALKING

Breakfast
1 slice whole-grain bread
1 T. natural peanut butter
1 T. natural fruit spread
Skinny latte or hot green tea

Fat-Blast Snack
1 low-fat cheese stick
20 grapes

Lunch
Tasty Tuna Delight
Fat-Blast Garden Mix or 7-Layer Salad (topped with Tasty Tuna Delight)

Fat-Blast Snack
2 oz. sliced turkey breast, rolled up with 2 asparagus spears,
¼ cup red pepper, dipped in mustard

Dinner
Caesar salad with 1 slice avocado and 1 T. dressing of choice
4 oz. grilled chicken with 2 t. pesto
Roasted vegetables: 1 cup cauliflower, 1 cup eggplant, topped with
½ oz. goat cheese

 LOWER YOUR BLOOD PRESSURE

If you have high blood pressure, try lowering your intake of sodium. Cook with fresh foods instead of processed or canned. Avoid using extra salt, and go light on condiments like ketchup or soy sauce. Using whole foods will also help you maintain a healthy weight, which aids in blood-pressure control. If you smoke, set your mind and body to quitting. And finally, limit the amount of alcohol you drink.

DAY 6

CALORIES: 1240

WORKOUT: STRETCHES AND INTERVAL WALKING

Breakfast
Egg white omelet
Add:
2 oz smoked salmon
1 t. capers, 1 t. diced red onion, 2 slices tomato
1 veggie sausage or 1 nitrite-free turkey bacon slice

Fat-Blast Snack
Skinny latte or hot green tea
Teriyaki Edamame (½ cup)

Lunch
Vegetarian Chili
10 baked tortilla chips
2 T. grated low-fat cheese
2 T. guacamole
Salsa

Fat-Blast Snack
2 t. dark chocolate chips
⅛ cup chopped raw almonds

Dinner
Asian Slaw Mix
Add:
2 T. dry roasted peanuts
4 oz. grilled flank steak
Stir fry: 1 t. toasted sesame oil, ¼ cup broccoli, ¼ cup carrot, ¼ cup red pepper, ¼ cup onion, ¼ cup shitake mushrooms

DAY 7:
SUPER SPLURGE!

CALORIES: 1500 (INCLUDES YOUR SUPER SPLURGE!)

WORKOUT: FUN ACTIVITY

Breakfast (80 calories)
Fat-Blast Green Energizer Smoothie

Lunch (280 calories)
Fat-Blast Garden Mix with 4 oz. of chicken salad, and 20 grapes added to chicken salad

Dinner: Super Splurge
1140 calories left to splurge on!

 USE OLIVE OIL SPRAY

Keep olive oil cooking spray by the stove, instead of using butter or margarine. Using this cooking spray (just a few sprays, please!) can cut out hundreds of calories from each dish you prepare.

DAY 8

CALORIES: 1100

WORKOUT: STRETCHES AND INTERVAL WALKING

Breakfast
Fat-Blast Fruit Energizer Smoothie

Fat-Blast Snack
Hot or cold green tea or skinny latte

Lunch
Bold Beet Salad on top of Fat-Blast Asian Slaw

Fat-Blast Snack
2 T. dark chocolate chips
⅛ cup chopped raw almonds

Dinner
Fat-Blast Salad Mix or 7-Layer Salad
Add:
Hearts of palm
1 T. Olive O Dressing
6 oz. sautéed shrimp mixed with ½ cup cooked quinoa, 1 t. dried
cherries, 2 T. chopped parsley, and 2 cloves roasted garlic

DAY 9

CALORIES: 1180

WORKOUT: STRETCHES AND 7-MINUTE SLIMMERS

Breakfast
White Corn Scramble
Sliced tomatoes
4 oz. orange juice

Fat-Blast Snack
Hot green tea

Lunch
Fat-Blast Asian Slaw
Add:
½ cup edamame
4 oz. grilled salmon
1 cup grilled bok choy

Fat-Blast Snack
1 sliced apple with 1 T. natural peanut butter

Dinner
Fat-Blast Bean Bowl
Grilled veggies: ½ cup zucchini, ½ cup red peppers, and ½ cup onions
2 T. shredded lettuce
2 T. grated low-fat cheese
2 T. guacamole
Salsa

DAY 10

CALORIES: 1240

WORKOUT: STRETCHES AND INTERVAL WALKING

Breakfast
1 cup plain, low-fat yogurt
½ cup berries: sliced strawberries, raspberries, blueberries, blackberries (choose one or several types)
1 T. crystallized ginger

Fat-Blast Snack
Skinny latte or hot green tea

Lunch
Flatbread Pizza

Fat-Blast Snack
½ cup carrots, ½ cup red pepper, ½ cup pea pods, dipped into ⅓ cup
hummus

Dinner
1 cup Super Vegetable Soup
Grilled chicken Caesar, 4 oz. grilled chicken breast
1 T. Olive O Dressing
Roasted vegetables: ½ cup zucchini, ½ cup peppers, 1 tomato, with
2 oz. goat cheese
½ cup fat-free frozen yogurt

★ FREE FOODS

If you're looking for "free foods" that won't disturb your weight loss, check this out. You can eat any vegetable "for free" except for corn and acorn or butternut squash. Legumes are not included because they are not vegetables. Fill up on vegetables like radishes, red and yellow peppers, chili peppers, snap peas, jicama, cherry tomatoes, green beans, and broccoli. You can dip them in salsa, a little ranch dressing, oil and vinegar, or sprinkle with spices like cayenne, seasoned salt, and cumin. You can always dip them in hummus, but that will add some extra carb calories. One very-low-calorie "free food" is cauliflower. I like to take cauliflower florets and dip them in cocktail sauce. It's amazing how this combination tastes like shrimp cocktail for less than ¼ of the calories.

Here are other free foods you'll love:

► Vegetable soup (select low-sodium and all-vegetable with broth. Make sure there are no added beans and pasta.)

► Crispy Kale (see page 206)

► Chicken Lettuce Wraps without chicken (page 186)

► Zesty Zucchini (go lighter on the cheese) (page 202)

► Teriyaki Edamame (page 130)

► Any veggie stir-fry

► Fat-Blast Garden Mix (page 189) or Fat-Blast Asian Slaw (page 190) with 1 T. dressing

► Fat-Blast Green Energizer Smoothie (page 191)

► Jicama Salad (page 197)

DAY 11

CALORIES: 1150

WORKOUT: STRETCHES AND 7-MINUTE SLIMMERS

Breakfast

3 egg whites
2 oz. smoked salmon or 2 oz. low-fat cheese
Capers, diced red onion, sliced tomatoes, parsley
4 oz. orange juice

Fat-Blast Snack

Teriyaki Edamame (½ cup)

Lunch

Tasty Tuna Delight
Fat-Blast Garden Mix or 7-Layer Salad (top with Tasty Tuna Delight)
Cut up: ½ cup carrots and ½ cup red pepper, dip in ¼ cup low-fat cottage cheese with pressed garlic, chives, and parsley

Fat-Blast Snack

1 small banana
Hot green tea

Dinner

Fat-Blast Asian Slaw
3 oz. loin lamb chops
Stir fry: ½ bok choy, ½ cup shitake mushrooms, ¼ cup shallots, parsley, 1 t. sesame oil

DAY 12

CALORIES: 1090

WORKOUT: STRETCHES AND INTERVAL WALKING

Breakfast
My Favorite Hot Cereal
Skinny latte

Fat-Blast Snack
½ grapefruit
2 T. chopped pecans

Lunch
Fat-Blast Garden Mix or 7-Layer Salad
Add:
½ cup egg salad (2 eggs, 1 T. light mayo)
5 whole-grain crackers

Fat-Blast Snack
Hot green tea

Dinner
1 cup Luscious Lentil Soup
1 cup spaghetti squash with ½ cup tomato sauce and pressed garlic
and 2 T. Parmesan cheese
3 oz. turkey burger (no bun)
Crispy Kale

DAY 13

CALORIES: 1270

WORKOUT: STRETCHES AND 7-MINUTE SLIMMERS

Breakfast

½ whole-wheat bagel
2 T. low-fat cream cheese
2 oz. smoked salmon
1 t. capers, 1 t. diced red onion, 1 slice tomato
½ grapefruit

Lunch

1 cup Super Veggie Soup
Chicken lettuce wraps

Fat-Blast Snack

1 apple with 1 T. natural peanut butter
Hot tea or skinny latte

Dinner

Fat-Blast Garden Mix or 7-Layer Salad with 1 T. choice of dressing
Vegetarian Chili
10 tortilla chips
2 T. grated low-fat cheese
2 T. guacamole
Salsa

DAY 14:
SUPER SPLURGE!

CALORIES: 1500 (INCLUDES YOUR SUPER SPLURGE!)

WORKOUT: FUN ACTIVITY

Breakfast (80 calories)
Fat-Blast Green Energizer Smoothie

Lunch (280 calories)
Fat-Blast Garden Mix with 4 oz. of chicken salad
20 grapes added to chicken salad

Dinner: Super Splurge
1140 calories left to splurge on!

 TOP 7 SKINNY PROTEIN SOURCES

1. Fish

2. Eggs (egg whites, egg substitutes)

3. Soy products

4. Legumes

5. Low-fat dairy products

6. Nuts, seeds, and soy nuts

7. Peanut butter and nut butters

DAY 15

CALORIES: 1190

WORKOUT: STRETCHES AND INTERVAL WALKING

Breakfast

Egg-white omelet

Add:

2 oz. smoked salmon

Capers, diced red onion, sliced tomato

1 veggie sausage or 1 slice nitrite free turkey bacon slice

Fat-Blast Snack

Hot green tea

Lunch

Fat-Blast Bean Bowl

Grilled veggies: ½ cup zucchini, ½ cup peppers, and ½ cup onions

2 T. shredded lettuce

2 T. grated low-fat cheese

2 T. guacamole

Salsa

Fat-Blast Snack

1 plum

2 T. roasted pumpkin seeds

Dinner

1 cup Super Veggie Soup

Fish or Shrimp Tacos

Crispy Kale

DAY 16

CALORIES: 1170

WORKOUT: STRETCHES AND 7-MINUTE SLIMMERS

Breakfast
Favorite Hot Cereal
4 oz. orange juice

Fat-Blast Snack
20 grapes
⅛ cup chopped raw walnuts

Lunch
Bold Beet Salad
Fat-Blast Garden Mix (topped with Bold Beet Salad)

Fat-Blast Snack
1 small carton of yogurt (90 calories)
1 T. ground chia seeds

Dinner
Fat-Blast Garden Mix or 7-Layer Salad
Add:
½ cup hearts of palm
1 T. Olive O Dressing
4 oz. sautéed tilapia or grilled salmon
Zesty Zucchini
Roasted vegetables: 1 tomato, 1 bulb fennel, ¼ cup black olives, and ½ cup sliced artichoke hearts

DAY 17

CALORIES: 1120

WORKOUT: STRETCHES AND INTERVAL WALKING

Breakfast
Fat-Blast Fruit Energizer Smoothie

Fat-Blast Snack
2 T. dark chocolate chips
¼ cup raw walnuts

Lunch
Tasty Tuna Delight Sandwich on 2 slices whole-grain bread
Crispy cut up veggies dipped in ¼ cup low-fat cottage cheese with
added parsley, chives, pressed garlic, seasoned salt

Fat-Blast Snack
Skinny latte or hot green tea
2 oz. sliced turkey breast, rolled up with 2 asparagus spears, ¼ cup
red pepper, dipped in mustard

Dinner
Fat-Blast Garden Mix or 7-Layer Salad
1 T. dressing of choice
Flatbread Pizza

 BEANS FILL YOU UP...NOT OUT

Beans are naturally low in fat and calories and high in fiber and protein. Just ½ cup of beans has 20 to 120 calories, 2 to 5 grams of fiber,
and 2 to 11 grams of protein!

DAY 18

CALORIES: 1250

WORKOUT: STRETCHES AND 7-MINUTE SLIMMERS

Breakfast

2 eggs: hard boiled, poached, scrambled, or 3-egg-white omelet
2 T. grated low-fat cheese
½ bag washed spinach leaves added to eggs
½ grapefruit

Lunch

1 cup Super Veggie Soup
Chicken lettuce wraps

Fat-Blast Snack

Hot green tea or skinny latte
2 T. roasted pumpkin seeds
1 apple

Dinner

Fat-Blast Asian Slaw

Add:
1 can water chestnuts
1 T. dried cranberries
½ cup edamame
3 oz. loin lamb chops
1 small medium potato
Roasted vegetables: 1 cup cauliflower, 1 cup eggplant

DAY 19

CALORIES: 1230

WORKOUT: STRETCHES AND INTERVAL WALKING

Breakfast
Fat-Blast Green Energizer Smoothie

Fat-Blast Snack
1 small carton of yogurt (90 calories)
1 T. chia seeds
Hot green tea

Lunch
Fat-Blast Garden Mix
Add:
¼ cup canned kidney or white beans
1 hard-boiled egg
1 T. Olive O Dressing
4 oz. beef, turkey, or veggie burger (no bun)

Fat-Blast Snack
1 T. pistachios
3 dates

Dinner
1 cup Luscious Lentil Soup
Vegan Stir Fry
Add:
3 oz. tofu (or 3 oz. chicken or steak)
Stir fry: 2 asparagus spears, ½ cup onions, ½ cup red pepper, ½ cup pea pods
1 t. red pepper flakes, 1 t. toasted sesame oil
½ cup frozen yogurt

DAY 20

CALORIES: 1120

WORKOUT: STRETCHES AND 7-MINUTE SLIMMERS

Breakfast
Skinny French Toast
Top with: ¾ cup blueberries. 1 t. maple syrup
1 slice turkey bacon (nitrite free)

Fat-Blast Snack
Skinny latte or hot green tea

Lunch
Bold Beet Salad
Fat-Blast Garden Mix (topped with Bold Beet Salad)
3 whole-grain crackers

Fat-Blast Snack
Sliced turkey breast rolls, dipped in mustard, with sliced cucumbers

Dinner
Fat-Blast Garden Mix or 7-Layer Salad
Add:
1 cup hearts of palm, sliced
1 T. dressing of choice
Vegetarian Chili
Top with: 3 T. grated low-fat cheese, 2 slices avocado, salsa

DAY 21:
SUPER SPLURGE!

CALORIES: 1500 (INCLUDES YOUR SUPER SPLURGE!)

WORKOUT: FUN ACTIVITY

Breakfast (80 calories)

Fat-Blast Green Energizer Smoothie

Lunch (280 calories)

Fat-Blast Garden Mix with 4 oz. of chicken salad and 20 grapes added to chicken salad

Dinner: Super Splurge

1140 calories left to splurge on!

CHAPTER 11

THE 7-DAY FAT-BLAST DIET AND WORKOUT: LEVEL 2

*Draw on your inner strength and
determination to stay the course!*

—*Denise*

You can stay on Level 2 for as long as you need to lose weight.

COMMITMENT Continue the Calorie Confusion as you trick your metabolism to boost fat loss. Also continue the Metabolism Confusion with the Interval Walking, stretches, and 7-Minute Slimmers strengthening exercises. By changing the number of calories you eat every few days and how you exercise, your metabolism will stay supercharged and the pounds will drop fast! Still allow for your Super Splurge every 7 days so you don't feel deprived. Develop healthy eating habits as you reintroduce the foods you love into your diet and focus on the exercises and activities you enjoy.

Once you have gone through all the sample menus for 5 weeks, go back and checkmark your favorite menus. Now create your own Level 2 diet as you continue this plan. Be sure to vary the calorie count of the menus for 7 days to include the following amounts for each week until you meet your weight goal:

Select 2 menus that are approximately 1100 calories.

Select 2 menus that are around 1200 calories.

Select 2 menus that are 1300 calories.

Select 1 Super Splurge menu that is around 1500-calories total (this is the same Super Splurge each week).

By varying the calorie counts every 2 days, you'll confuse your metabolism and burn calories at a faster pace!

 ### 5 MORE DAILY BLITZES FOR YOU HIGH-FLYERS!

Here are 5 more blitzes for women who want to take it up a notch!

► **Squeeze that butt.** Do it in the elevator, as you are walking down the aisles of a grocery store, and while you are waiting in line at the bank. No one will know—and it is so effective!

► **Work those legs.** Try doing leg lifts at your desk or squats while you brush your teeth at night.

► **Tuck that tummy.** Instead of just sitting in front of the TV for the entire show, get on the floor and do some crunches at every commercial break.

► **Relieve some tension.** Sitting hunched over a desk or staring at a computer for 8 hours a day can cause tension in your upper body, specifically your neck, back, and shoulders. Stretching is a good way to relieve that tension and get tight muscles to relax. Once an hour, do my 3 daily stretches on page 51 and give those muscles a break.

► **Do some phone squats.** Instead of sitting in a chair while you chat, ditch the chair and do some wall sits. Pretend you're sitting in a chair, with your back up against a wall and your knees bent at a 45 to 90 degree angle. Either hold the pose for as long as you can, or try holding it for 60 seconds, then pace for 60 seconds and repeat.

DAY 22

CALORIES: 1130

WORKOUT: STRETCHES AND INTERVAL WALKING

Breakfast
White Corn Scramble
Sliced tomatoes
2 slices turkey bacon
½ grapefruit

Lunch
Tuna Delight
Fat-Blast Garden Mix (topped with Tuna Delight)
1 corn tortilla with 2 T. low-fat grated cheese, 1 slice avocado
Salsa

Fat-Blast Snack
2 oz. sliced turkey, rolled up with asparagus, red pepper, and dipped in mustard
Hot green tea or skinny latte

Dinner
Caesar salad with:
1 T. dressing of choice
4 oz. grilled chicken, fish, or steak
3 roasted red potatoes
1 cup spaghetti squash with ½ cup tomato sauce and pressed garlic and 2 T. Parmesan cheese

DAY 23

CALORIES: 1350

WORKOUT: STRETCHES AND 7-MINUTE SLIMMERS

Breakfast
1 slice whole-grain bread
1 T. natural peanut butter
1 T. natural fruit spread
Skinny latte or hot green tea

Fat-Blast Snack
1 plum
⅛ cup chopped raw walnuts

Lunch
Fat-Blast Garden Mix
Add:
½ cup kidney beans
3 oz. of turkey breast
1 slice of avocado

Fat-Blast Snack
½ cup baby carrots, ½ red pepper, ½ cup cucumber slices, dipped in ¼ cup low-fat cottage cheese mixed with chives, pressed garlic, and fresh chopped basil

Dinner
Sliced tomato, 2 oz. fresh mozzarella, fresh basil, diced red onion
4 oz. roasted chicken
½ baked sweet potato with cinnamon
Roasted vegetables: 1 cup cauliflower, 1 fennel bulb, and 6 asparagus spears with pressed garlic

DAY 24

CALORIES: 1570

WORKOUT: STRETCHES AND INTERVAL WALKING

Breakfast
3-egg-white omelet with spinach (½ bag washed) and
2 T. feta cheese
Salsa

Fat-Blast Snack
Tangerine
Hot green tea

Lunch
1 turkey sandwich on 2 slices whole-wheat bread with mustard,
topped with lots of fresh veggies and pickle spear
1 cup carrots, 1 sliced cucumber dipped in ⅓ cup hummus

Fat-Blast Snack
Hot green tea
2 squares dark chocolate

Dinner
Caesar salad with 1 T. dressing of choice
¾ cup pasta with tomato sauce and 2 T. Parmesan cheese
Add:
4 oz. shrimp
Crispy Kale

 TAKE IT UP A NOTCH ON THE TREADMILL

Interval training is all about changing the level of intensity by
changing the speed (faster and slower) as well as the incline of the
treadmill. Both are individually effective, but combining the 2 in a
single workout on the treadmill is the best way to get results!

DAY 25

CALORIES: 1150

WORKOUT: STRETCHES AND 7-MINUTE SLIMMERS

Breakfast

1 cup plain low-fat yogurt
1 cup berries: sliced strawberries, raspberries, blueberries, blackberries (choose one or several types)
1 T. toasted, chopped walnuts
1 T. crystallized ginger

Fat-Blast Snack

Skinny latte or hot green tea

Lunch

Fat-Blast Garden Mix

Add:
Roasted red peppers
2 T. sunflower seeds
3 oz. roast turkey breast or grilled salmon

Fat-Blast Snack

4 stalks of celery
1 T. natural peanut butter

Dinner

1 cup Super Vegetable Soup
Chicken Lettuce Wraps

Add:
⅓ cup brown rice

DAY 26

CALORIES: 1150

WORKOUT: STRETCHES AND INTERVAL WALKING

Breakfast

Fat-Blast Fruit Energizer Smoothie

Fat-Blast Snack

Skinny latte or hot green tea
Apple with 1 T. peanut butter

Lunch

Vegetarian chili
10 baked tortilla chips
2 T. grated low-fat cheese
2 T. guacamole
Salsa
Put atop Fat-Blast Garden Mix, if desired

Fat-Blast Snack

2 T. dark chocolate chips
⅛ cup chopped raw almonds

Dinner

Fat-Blast Asian Slaw
4 oz. grilled flank steak
Stir fry: ½ cup broccoli, ½ cup carrots, ½ cup red pepper, ¼ cup
onions, ¼ cup shitake mushrooms, 1 t. sesame oil

DAY 27

CALORIES: 1220

WORKOUT: STRETCHES AND 7-MINUTE SLIMMERS

Breakfast
My Favorite Hot Cereal
4 oz. orange juice

Fat-Blast Snack
1 apple
⅛ cup chopped raw walnuts

Lunch
Bold Beet Salad
Fat-Blast Garden Mix (topped with Bold Beet Salad)

Fat-Blast Snack
1 small carton of yogurt (90 calories)
2 T. chia seeds

Dinner
Fat-Blast Garden Mix or 7-Layer Salad
Add:
Hearts of palm
1 T. Olive O Dressing
4 oz. grilled chicken
Zesty Zucchini
Roasted vegetables: 1 tomato, 1 fennel bulb, 2 T. black olives, ½ cup artichoke hearts

DAY 28:
SUPER SPLURGE!

CALORIES: 1500 (INCLUDES YOUR SUPER SPLURGE!)

WORKOUT: FUN ACTIVITY

Breakfast (80 calories)

Fat-Blast Green Energizer Smoothie

Lunch (280 calories)

Fat-Blast Garden Mix with 4 oz. of chicken salad
20 grapes added to chicken salad

Dinner: Super Splurge

1140 calories left to splurge on!

HIGH-INTENSITY EXERCISES FOR THOSE WHO ARE AEROBICALLY FIT

- ▶ Aerobics (high-impact)
- ▶ Basketball
- ▶ Biking (hills)
- ▶ Dancing (fast)
- ▶ Hiking
- ▶ Jogging
- ▶ Jumping rope
- ▶ Karate

- ▶ Kick boxing
- ▶ Rollerblading
- ▶ Running
- ▶ Soccer
- ▶ Spinning (ultra-intensity indoor cycling)
- ▶ Swimming (fast)
- ▶ Tennis (singles)

DAY 29

CALORIES: 1170

WORKOUT: STRETCHES AND INTERVAL WALKING

Breakfast

Egg-white omelet

Add:

2 oz. smoked salmon

1 oz. goat cheese

Capers, diced red onion, sliced tomato

1 veggie sausage or 1 slice nitrite free turkey bacon slice

Fat-Blast Snack

Hot green tea

Lunch

Fat-Blast Bean Bowl

Fat-Blast Snack

1 plum

2 T. roasted pumpkin seeds

Dinner

1 cup Super Veggie Soup

Fish or Shrimp Tacos

Add:

2 T chopped avocado

Jicama Salad

Crispy Kale

DAY 30

CALORIES: 1420

WORKOUT: STRETCHES AND 7-MINUTE SLIMMERS

BREAKFAST

My Favorite Hot Cereal
4 oz. orange juice

Fat-Blast Snack

20 grapes
⅛ cup chopped raw walnuts

Lunch

Fat-Blast Garden Mix or 7-Layer Salad with 1 T. choice of dressing
4 oz. turkey burger with grilled onions and mushrooms (no bun)

Fat-Blast Snack

1 small carton of yogurt (90 calories)
1 T. chia seeds

Dinner

Fat-Blast Garden Mix
Add:
Hearts of palm
1 T. Olive O Dressing
4 oz. flank steak or filet
Zesty Zucchini
1 medium Idaho potato, baked

DAY 31

CALORIES: 1340

WORKOUT: STRETCHES AND INTERVAL WALKING

Breakfast
Fat-Blast Fruit Energizer Smoothie

Fat-Blast Snack
2 t. dark chocolate chips
¼ cup raw walnuts

Lunc
Tasty Tuna Delight on 2 slices whole-wheat bread with lettuce and tomato (can substitute 4 oz. chicken salad or 4 oz. egg salad for tuna)
10 baked tortilla chips
1 cup carrots, 1 cup broccoli florets cut up dipped in ⅔ cup hummus

Fat-Blast Snack
Teriyaki Edamame (½ cup)

Dinner
Fat-Blast Garden Mix
2 T. Olive O Dressing
Flatbread Pizza

DAY 32

CALORIES: 1250

WORKOUT: STRETCHES AND 7-MINUTE SLIMMERS

Breakfast
2 eggs: hardboiled, poached, scrambled, or 3-egg-white omelet
2 T. grated low-fat cheese
½ bag of washed spinach leaves
½ grapefruit

Fat-Blast Snack
1 apple

Lunch
1 cup Super Veggie Soup
Chicken lettuce wraps
Add: ⅓ cup brown rice

Fat-Blast Snack
Hot green tea or skinny latte
2 T. roasted pumpkin seeds

Dinner
Fat-Blast Asian Slaw
Add:
1 can water chestnuts
1 T. dried cranberries
¼ cup edamame
3 oz. loin lamb chops
Roasted vegetables: 1 cup broccoli, 1 cup eggplant

DAY 33

CALORIES: 1250

WORKOUT: STRETCHES AND INTERVAL WALKING

Breakfast

Fat-Blast Green Energizer Smoothie

Fat-Blast Snack

1 small carton of yogurt (90 calories)
1 T. chia seeds
Hot green tea

Lunch

Fat-Blast Garden Mix

Add:

¼ cup white beans cooked
1 hard-boiled egg
1 T. Olive O Dressing
4 oz. turkey burger

Fat-Blast Snack

½ cup frozen yogurt

Dinner

1 cup Luscious Lentil Soup
Vegan Stir Fry

Add:

3 oz. tofu (or 3 oz. chicken)
½ cup brown rice
Stir fry: 4 asparagus spears, ¼ cup onions, 1 red pepper, ½ cup pea
pods, 1 t. sesame oil, red pepper flakes to taste

DAY 34

CALORIES: 1150

WORKOUT: STRETCHES AND 7-MINUTE SLIMMERS

BREAKFAST

Skinny French Toast
Top with:
¾ cup blueberries
1 t. maple syrup
2 slices turkey bacon (nitrite free)

Fat-Blast Snack

Skinny latte or hot green tea

Lunch

Bold Beet Salad
Fat-Blast Garden Mix (topped with Bold Beet Salad)

Fat-Blast Snack

3 oz. sliced turkey breast, dipped in spicy mustard, with 1 cup sliced
red peppers

Dinner

Fat-Blast Garden Mix or 7-Layer Salad
Add:
Hearts of palm
Artichoke hearts
1 T. Olive O Dressing
Vegetarian Chili
Top with: 2 T. avocado, salsa

DAY 35:
SUPER SPLURGE!

CALORIES: 1500 (INCLUDES YOUR SUPER SPLURGE!)

WORKOUT: FUN ACTIVITY

Breakfast (80 calories)
Fat-Blast Green Energizer Smoothie

Lunch (280 calories)
Fat-Blast Garden Mix with 4 oz. of chicken salad
20 grapes added to chicken salad

Dinner: Super Splurge
1140 calories left to splurge on!

 LIFT AND TIGHTEN THE BUTT

The butt can sag, so it is a critical target zone! One excellent exercise that will help lift and tone your rear is the squat. Stand with your feet hip width apart, bend your knees, and lower your hips until your thighs are parallel to the ground, making sure your knees don't go past your toes, then use your glutes to push back into the standing position. If squats bother your knees, try standing leg lifts. Alternate lifting each leg out behind you, again using your glutes to both power and control the move. Either of these tush toners can be done as you get ready for work or wash up the dishes. Hey, you can exercise anytime, anywhere!

TRAIN LIKE A SUPERSTAR!

▶ **Set a goal.** Watching athletes play football, baseball, or any team sport is a perfect reminder of how important setting a goal is to achieving results. Having a concrete goal to work toward will keep you on track, even on the days you feel like skipping a workout.

▶ **Train with a team.** Watching athletes on any team cheer each other on through the good moments and bad is motivating and a team of your own will do the same for you! Recruit a walking buddy or a group of colleagues who want to lose weight, and start cheering each other along.

▶ **Find an activity you love.** All athletes are passionate about their sport, which keeps them motivated even when workouts are tough or an injury causes a setback. Make exercise enjoyable by finding an activity you love to do! Dancing, tennis, walking on the beach—they all count!

▶ **Fuel up.** If anyone knows the importance of proper nutrition, it is athletes. Feeding their bodies with healthy foods is crucial for repairing muscles and keeping energy up. Follow their lead, and fill your own diet with lots of fruits, veggies, whole grains, and lean protein.

▶ **Forgive yourself for slip ups.** Everyone has off days, even the all-stars. When injuries or mistakes during competition occur, true athletes get right back up and keep going. Let it inspire you to never give up or give in on *your* dreams.

CHAPTER 12

SKINNY RECIPES

Get creative and express yourself in the kitchen!
Empower yourself to find ways to enjoy the
healthiest foods.

—Denise

These Skinny Recipes for my 7-Day Fat-Blast Diet are made with the healing foods and nutrients discussed throughout the book. For example, antioxidants and phytochemicals found in fruits and vegetables are important to keep your immune system working efficiently and to prevent illness. Soy and dairy products keep your bones and teeth strong and may boost your metabolism to help you lose weight faster. Omega-3 fatty acids found in salmon, tuna fish, and olive oil help reduce inflammation—the root of many chronic diseases. If you are someone who wants to make every calorie count nutritionally, these recipes will help you to get healthier with the added side effect of slimming down, too!

CHICKEN LETTUCE WRAPS

I love lettuce wraps; Asian flavors with just a few calories. These are so quick and easy. They make a perfect dinner on a night when you are too tired to cook.

SERVES: 4
EACH SERVING: 150 calories

INGREDIENTS:

8 oz. steamed chicken breasts, diced (or 1 block firm tofu)

1 can water chestnuts, sliced (8 oz.)

1 can bamboo shoots, diced (8 oz.)

½ cup diced scallions

2 cloves garlic, finely chopped

¼ cup finely chopped cilantro

1 T. low-sodium soy sauce

1 T. rice vinegar

1 T. sesame oil

1 t. chili paste

8 large iceberg lettuce leaves, separated, washed, and patted dry

DIRECTIONS:

Steam chicken breasts in a steamer. When cooled, dice into small pieces. Or if using tofu, follow the directions on the package for cooking. Place chicken into a bowl. Add water chestnuts, bamboo shoots, scallions, garlic, and cilantro. Mix together soy sauce, rice vinegar, sesame oil, and chili paste. Add soy sauce mixture to chicken. Stir well. Divide the chicken mixture evenly onto the 8 lettuce leaves. Serve 2 leaves on each plate.

FLATBREAD PIZZA

My delicious pizza hits the spot when you are fat-blasting. Instead of a thick crust, this thin whole-wheat wrap makes a delicious base for all kinds of flatbread pizzas. Try new flavors by mixing and matching vegetables, proteins, and spices. These are good for either lunch or dinner.

SERVES: 2
EACH SERVING: 240 calories

INGREDIENTS:

2 whole-wheat, whole-grain, sprouted-wheat, or gluten-free wraps or tortillas (100 calories each)

1 large tomato, sliced

4 canned artichoke hearts packed in water, drained, and cut in half

6 olives, drained and sliced

½ cup diced onions

¼ cup low-fat grated cheese

2 T. jarred pizza sauce

DIRECTIONS:

Preheat oven to 350°. Lay both tortillas on a large baking sheet. Spread pizza sauce thinly over the wraps or tortillas. Divide the tomato slices, artichokes halves, sliced olives, and diced onions evenly between the 2 pizzas. Place in oven for 8 minutes or until wraps start to get crispy.
Add grated cheese and place back in the oven for 3 minutes or until melted. Remove from oven. Place on a plate and eat while warm.

SKINNY FRENCH TOAST

For Sunday brunch, a holiday treat, or anytime you need comfort food in the morning! Easy to make and delicious.

SERVES: 4
EACH SERVING: 225

INGREDIENTS:

4 slices whole-grain, whole-wheat, or gluten-free bread

4 eggs, yolks separated, or ½ cup of egg whites from a carton

1 t. cinnamon

1 t. olive oil or olive oil spray to coat pan

½ cup blueberries, strawberries, or raspberries

1 T. maple syrup

DIRECTIONS:

In a large frying pan, add olive oil, or spray with oil mist. Use 1 whole egg and 3 egg whites, tossing out the extra yolks, or ½ cup egg whites from a carton. Place in bowl and beat well. Add cinnamon to egg mixture, stir well. Place egg mixture in a shallow bowl. Place frying pan on stove and turn heat on to medium. Dip each piece of bread into the egg mixture, coating both sides. Then place into hot pan. Cook bread on both sides until egg is golden. If toast is sticking, add more spray. Remove slices from pan, place each on a plate, and top with sliced fruit and a drizzle of real maple syrup.

FAT-BLAST GARDEN MIX

This green mixture is a staple of the 7-Day Fat-Blast diet. This can be made ahead and kept in the refrigerator. Having this on hand will ensure that you fill up on plenty of low-calorie, highly nutritious greens. No excuses needed! If you don't like the ones I suggest, add the ones you like. Wash all vegetables prior to cutting. Store in an airtight container or plastic bag.

SERVES: 6
EACH SERVING: 60 calories

INGREDIENTS:

1 cup each arugula, romaine, spinach, or mixed packaged greens

3 carrots, chopped

3 large tomatoes, diced (keep these separate until just prior to serving or the mix will get soggy)

1 large bulb fennel, diced (discard tops)

1 cup fresh chopped basil leaves

1 large red or white onion, diced

1 large cucumber diced

DIRECTIONS:

Wash greens and spin-dry or dry between paper towels. Place in a large bowl. Add all other vegetables, except tomatoes, and mix well. Store in an airtight container in the refrigerator. Place tomatoes in a separate covered bowl. Before serving, add tomatoes. Remember, though, once you've washed vegetables, they lose their freshness faster, so make sure you eat them within 1 or 2 days of washing.

FAT-BLAST ASIAN SLAW

Cool and refreshing, this Asian slaw can be eaten any time of day. Cabbage is very high in sulfur compounds, which are thought to help prevent certain types of cancers. Use this slaw as a salad base for variety and crunch. Like the Garden Mix, prepare a large amount to have on hand. This mixture can be substituted for the Garden Mix if you like. This needs no added dressing since the dressing is already mixed in.

SERVES: 6
EACH SERVING: 100 calories

INGREDIENTS:

1 large Chinese cabbage

1 large green cabbage

8 scallions, washed and tips trimmed

1 large red onion

2 T. fresh diced ginger, peeled

½ cup rice vinegar

2 T. low-sodium soy sauce

2 T. toasted sesame oil

1 t. dried red pepper flakes or 1 t. chili paste

DIRECTIONS:

Core both cabbages. Using a large knife, slice cabbages into thin slices, then dice with knife. Finely chop scallions. Dice red onion. Dice ginger. Mix the following together in a separate bowl: rice vinegar, soy sauce, toasted sesame seed oil, and red pepper or chili paste. Pour vinegar mixture over vegetable slaw and mix well. Store in an air-tight container.

FAT-BLAST GREEN ENERGIZER SMOOTHIE

Smoothies make a refreshing and filling breakfast. Whether you're in a hurry or just in the mood for a frothy drink, smoothies also make a great meal replacement. You can mix and match the fruits and greens. If you don't like what I like, use the fruits and vegetables that you desire. Wash greens well because they can be gritty.

SERVES: 2
EACH SERVING: 80 calories

INGREDIENTS:

8 oz. canned or fresh pineapple juice or 1 cup fresh pineapple (You can substitute or add in papaya, mango, or kiwi for a new fun flavor)

1 large handful of fresh kale (1½ cups)

1 large handful of fresh spinach (1½ cups)

1 T. chopped fresh ginger root

Add more water if needed

Ice cubes for froth

DIRECTIONS:

Place all ingredients in a high-powered blender. Mix until well blended. Pour into a glass. (Store unused portion in a covered glass in the refrigerator or in a thermos. Take leftovers to work for a mid-morning snack.)

FAT-BLAST FRUIT ENERGIZER SMOOTHIE

This smoothie is yogurt-based, giving you a dose of probiotics. Fresh or frozen fruit can be used. Like the Fat-Blast Green Energizer Smoothie, this fruit smoothie can be used as a meal replacement or a snack. Use these fruits or ones you love.

SERVES: 2
EACH SERVING: 120 calories

INGREDIENTS:

1 cup plain yogurt

½ banana

1 cup frozen mixed mango, strawberry, or blueberries

1 t. green tea extract (or brew a cup of green tea and add to smoothie with an extra cup of ice to keep the smoothie consistency perfect)

1 T. cocoa powder (optional for chocolate lovers.)

Ice cubes for froth

Optional: Add whey or hemp protein powder to fill you up

DIRECTIONS:

Place yogurt, banana, and frozen and/or fresh fruit into blender. Add green tea extract or green tea. Optional: Add cocoa powder and/or sweetener. Add ice cubes. Blend well. Pour into glass. Store extra in thermos or covered glass in refrigerator.

TASTY TUNA DELIGHT

This tangy tuna dish is easy to make and certain to delight. Use water-packed white albacore tuna. Made ahead, you can take it for lunch or toss it onto either the Fat-Blast Garden Mix or Fat-Blast Asian Slaw for a filling meal. Eat it with raw vegetables for a snack in the late afternoon. You can wrap the tuna in a lettuce leaf or add a slice of low-fat cheese for a tuna melt!

SERVES: 4
EACH SERVING: 80 calories

INGREDIENTS:

1 large can albacore, water-packed tuna, drained (6 oz.)

4 T. red wine vinegar

4 T. capers

2 T. lemon juice

¼ cup chopped parsley

2 cloves pressed garlic

Salt and pepper to taste

DIRECTIONS:

Open tuna and drain out water. Place in large bowl and separate with a fork. In a separate bowl, mix together vinegar, capers, lemon juice, chopped parsley, and garlic. Add vinegar mixture to tuna and stir well. Add to Fat-Blast Garden Mix or Fat-Blast Asian Slaw. Or you can use as an antipasto with chopped fresh vegetables, sliced avocado, and roasted red peppers. Store remaining mixture in covered container in the refrigerator.

FAT-BLAST BEAN BOWL

Black beans are an excellent source of fiber, so they really give an added punch to the chicken and veggies here. You can also use this as a dip for whole-grain chips or wrap it in a whole-grain tortilla.

SERVES: 4
EACH SERVING: 160 calories

INGREDIENTS:

4 oz. grilled chicken breast, diced

¼ cup grated low-fat cheese

1 cup black beans, canned (or cooked at home), liquid reserved

½ cup diced tomatoes

½ cup diced white onions

½ cup diced red, yellow, or orange pepper

1 cup salsa

1 t. olive oil

¼ cup chopped cilantro

1 lime

Optional: 1 t. cumin

DIRECTIONS:

Open and drain black beans in colander, saving a little of the liquid from the can. Once drained, place beans in a saucepan and warm on medium heat. Add the little bit of saved liquid. Add diced, grilled chicken breast to beans. In a separate pan, sauté pepper and onions in 1 t. olive oil. When translucent, add diced tomatoes and cook for 3 minutes. If you like cumin, add it with the tomatoes. When the beans and chicken are heated thoroughly, add them to the peppers, onions, and tomatoes. Divide into 4 servings and place in bowls. Top with each bowl with ¼ each of the cheese and cilantro. Squirt ½ a lime into each bowl for zest.

VEGETARIAN CHILI

Nothing says comfort food in the winter like a steaming bowl of chili. Feel free to play with the seasonings and suit it to the level of spiciness you crave. This is also a great meal for vegetarians, and to make it vegan, simply eliminate the cheese.

SERVES: 6
EACH SERVING: 70 calories

INGREDIENTS:

1 cup canned black, pinto, or kidney beans, with liquid

½ cup diced tomatoes, fresh or canned

1 cup tomato juice

2 jalapeno peppers, seeded and diced

½ cup diced yellow onions

½ cup diced peeled carrots

½ cup chopped cilantro

¼ cup low-fat grated cheese

1 t. cumin

1 t. salt

1 t. chili powder

1 t. garlic powder

Dash of cinnamon

DIRECTIONS:

Into a large soup pot, add 1 t. olive oil. Heat oil and add onions, carrots, cilantro, jalapeno peppers, tomatoes, cumin, cinnamon, salt, chili powder, and garlic powder. Stir well and cook until soft, about 10–15 minutes. Add tomato juice and beans. Cook another 10 minutes. Divide chili into bowls and top with grated cheese.

FISH OR SHRIMP TACOS

Fish or shrimp tacos made with soft corn tortillas bring Mexican flavor into your home throughout the year. If you don't like shrimp, you can substitute any fish. Salmon, halibut, and tilapia all work. Make sure to remove bones before serving. Shredded cabbage can be added to the tacos for added flavor.

SERVES: 2
EACH SERVING: 220 calories

INGREDIENTS:

4 soft corn tortillas

4 oz. cooked, shelled, deveined, and diced shrimp (or 4 oz. of white fish—I like tilapia!)

¼ cup diced, yellow onions

¼ cup chopped cilantro

¼ cup chopped tomatoes

1 t. olive oil

1 lime

Sprinkle of cayenne pepper

DIRECTIONS:

Preheat oven to 350°. On a baking sheet, spread out 4 corn tortillas. Put aside. Chop cooked shrimp into small pieces. In 1 t. olive oil, sauté shrimp, onions, cilantro, and tomatoes for about 5 minutes or until heated through. While heating shrimp mixture, place baking sheet with tortillas in oven for about 5 minutes until soft and moist. Watch carefully so they don't burn. Take out of oven and put 2 tortillas on each plate. When the shrimp mixture is heated through, divide it evenly between the 4 tortillas. Squirt with a dash of lime juice and cayenne.

JICAMA SALAD

Jicama is a large root that resembles a cross between a potato and a radish, but with a sweet juicy taste. It is a great accompaniment to any Mexican dish. Jicama is perfect for dipping into salsa or hummus. Sprinkled with lime juice and a little chili powder, jicama makes a refreshing midday snack.

SERVES: 4
EACH SERVING: 280 calories

INGREDIENTS:

1 large jicama root, washed

½ cup fresh-squeezed lime juice

2 cups fresh sliced mango

½ cup cilantro sprigs

Sprinkle of chili powder

½ cup dry-roasted peanuts, crushed

DIRECTIONS:

Peel the skin off the jicama with a knife or potato peeler. Slice the jicama and the mango into long narrow strips, about 1 inch long and ½ inch wide. Place mango and jicama into a bowl. Toss with fresh-squeezed lime juice and a sprinkle of chili powder. Divide into 4 servings and arrange on plates. Top with crushed, dry-roasted peanuts. Garnish with cilantro sprigs.

OLIVE O DRESSING

Olive oil is a healthy fat and has a wonderful flavor that brings out the fresh taste of salads. This dressing keeps in the refrigerator for weeks. Make a large portion and have it on hand for all your salads. Olive oil congeals when refrigerated. Let the jar of dressing sit in warm water for 30 seconds to loosen. Put remainder back in refrigerator. This is also a good marinade for grilled chicken or meats.

MAKES: 16 Servings
SERVING SIZE: 1 T.
EACH SERVING: 35 calories

INGREDIENTS:

¼ cup extra-virgin, cold-pressed olive oil

½ cup red wine vinegar

2 T. Dijon mustard

¼ freshly chopped basil leaves

2 T. balsamic vinegar

2 cloves garlic, pressed

Salt and freshly ground pepper to taste

DIRECTIONS:

Pour olive oil into a large glass jar with a tight-fitting lid. Add red wine and balsamic vinegars, mustard, garlic, and basil leaves. Place lid on jar. Shake well to mix all ingredients. Add salt and pepper to taste. Store in refrigerator.

LUSCIOUS LENTIL SOUP

Lentil soup is a family favorite. You can either cook your own lentils or use canned or precooked lentils in foil pouches, available at your favorite grocery store. Be adventurous and try red or yellow lentils.

SERVES: 6
EACH SERVING: 140 calories

INGREDIENTS:

6 cups low-fat, low-sodium chicken stock

2 cups canned lentils, cooked

¼ cup diced onions

2 cups raw spinach

2 celery stalks, diced

1 t. cumin

1 t. ground coriander

1½ large tomatoes chopped

2 cloves garlic, pressed

2 t. olive oil

Salt and pepper to taste

DIRECTIONS:

In a large soup pot, heat 2 t. olive oil and sauté carrots, onions, spinach, celery, cumin, garlic, and coriander until soft, about 10 minutes. Add chopped tomatoes and cook another 5 minutes. Mix well. Add chicken stock and lentils and bring to a boil. Quickly lower heat to a simmer. Cook for 10 minutes until heated through. Add salt and pepper to taste. Serve warm or reheat before serving.

7-LAYER SALAD

This 7-Layer Salad is the perfect accompaniment to any meal. It can stand alone as a delicious colorful salad or as the basis for many of my favorite salad stuffers. Simple to make and easy to store, this mouthwatering salad can be used interchangeably with the Fat-Blast Garden Mix. Both salads have 60 calories per serving.

SERVES: 6
EACH SERVING: 60 calories

INGREDIENTS:

3 cups fresh, baby spinach, washed

½ cup finely chopped carrots, peeled

2 tomatoes, finely chopped

1 yellow pepper, finely chopped

1 red pepper, finely chopped

1 cup celery, finely diced

¼ cup kidney or cannellini beans, well drained

¼ cup grated Parmesan cheese

DIRECTIONS:

Wash all vegetables well. Spin-dry spinach or place between paper towels to remove any moisture. Place in the bottom of a glass bowl. Peel carrots. Core peppers and remove seeds and gills. Chop carrots, tomatoes, peppers, and celery, making sure to keep them all separate. Next, layer beans over the spinach. Add carrots, tomatoes, yellow pepper, red pepper, and celery. Top with Parmesan cheese.

SUPER VEGETABLE SOUP

A bowl of liquid garden is how I would describe this hearty soup. Any kind of vegetable can be added for flavor and texture. This soup can be eaten any time of the day for a warm and filling snack or meal.

SERVES: 6
EACH SERVING: 70 calories

INGREDIENTS:

6 cups low-fat, low-sodium chicken stock

½ cup carrots, diced

½ green cabbage, sliced thin

½ cup parsnips, diced

½ cup yellow onions, diced

1 cup canned, diced tomatoes (do not drain liquid)

½ cup fresh basil leaves, chopped

2 cloves garlic, minced

1 t. olive oil

Salt and pepper to taste

Parsley sprigs for garnish

DIRECTIONS:

In a large soup pot, add olive oil and sauté carrots, cabbage, onions, parsnips, garlic, and basil leaves until soft. After 10 minutes, add canned tomatoes with liquid. Add chicken broth and simmer for 30 minutes. Serve warm in bowls. Top with parsley sprigs.

ZESTY ZUCCHINI

Zucchini is a versatile year-round vegetable that has a delicate flavor and a soft texture. Zucchini is delicious roasted and can add body and flavor to rice, pastas, breads, and cookies. Sliced raw, zucchini is a perfect accompaniment to fresh herb and vegetable dips. For another yummy version of my Zesty Zucchini recipe, you can add 2 tablespoons low-sodium tomato sauce and a sprinkle of low-fat mozzarella cheese for just 25 calories more!

SERVES: 4
EACH SERVING: 90 calories

INGREDIENTS:

4 medium-sized zucchinis

1 T. olive oil

2 T. pressed garlic

3 T. grated Parmesan cheese

Optional: For 25 extra calories, add 2 tbsp. low-sodium tomato sauce and a sprinkle of mozzarella cheese.

DIRECTIONS:

Preheat oven to broil. Wash and trim zucchini. Cut in half lengthwise. Place on a baking sheet with edges. Rub zucchini halves with olive oil. Sprinkle pressed garlic on top. Broil for 8 minutes until soft. Remove from broiler and sprinkle on Parmesan cheese. Return to broiler for 2 minutes or until cheese is melted and golden. Remove from oven and place 2 slices on each plate.

MY FAVORITE HOT CEREAL

Oat bran is the outer layer of an oat and is loaded with soluble fiber which helps keep your cholesterol levels in check. Oat bran makes a filling breakfast cereal, and when mixed with fresh fruit and nuts is a heavenly treat.

SERVES: 4
EACH SERVING: 90 calories

INGREDIENTS:

¼ cup oat bran

1 cup water

¾ cup fresh, washed blueberries

2 T. ground flaxseed

2 T. chopped walnuts

1 cup nonfat milk (optional)

DIRECTIONS:

Bring water to a boil in a saucepan. Add ¼ cup oat bran and 2 T. ground flaxseed. Stir well. Turn down the heat, cover, and let mixture cook for 5 minutes until it's the consistency of porridge. Remove from heat and place into bowls. Add walnuts, blueberries, and milk.

WHITE CORN OMELET

Eggs are full of protein, but the debate still rages as to whether or not you should eat the yolk or just the white. I recommend mostly whites, with a yolk or 2 here and there. However, whether you eat the entire egg, or just the white, eggs are a versatile food that can be eaten for breakfast, lunch, or dinner. Here's my favorite way to eat them.

SERVES: 2
EACH SERVING: 110 calories

INGREDIENTS:

4 egg whites, plus 1 yolk

4 T. fresh or frozen white corn

1½ cups fresh, washed spinach

2 T. chopped chives

3 T. chopped parsley

2 large tomatoes, diced

Olive oil spray

DIRECTIONS:

Break eggs into a large bowl, taking care to separate whites from yolks. Toss out the unused yolks. Beat egg mixture with a fork until blended. Add corn, spinach, chives, parsley, and diced tomatoes. Spray frying pan with olive oil spray and place over low heat. Add egg and vegetable mixture. Cook over medium-low heat until greens are wilted and eggs are done. Divide equally between 2 plates.

BOLD BEET SALAD

Beets are a bold vegetable, full of colorful plant antioxidants and blood-building iron. Beets' earthy flavors make them a perfect addition to any salad. Make sure you wear gloves when handling beets or your fingers will be temporarily stained red! Or purchase canned, sliced beets.

SERVES: 6
EACH SERVING: 160 calories

INGREDIENTS:

6 beets (2" in diameter), washed and trimmed

1 cup canned, cooked lentils

2 cups fresh, washed arugula

4 oz. crumbled goat cheese (optional)

1 t. olive oil

¼ cup fresh lemon juice

2 T. chopped fresh parsley

2 T. chopped fresh basil

Salt to taste

NOTE: To save time, you can buy pre-cooked beets and lentils at the grocery store that are ready to eat.

DIRECTIONS:

Wash beets thoroughly, removing stems and leaves. Trim off peel and rough areas. To roast: wrap beets in foil and roast in oven at 350 degrees for 45 minutes. To steam: place in steamer basket for 20 minutes or until tender. Once beets are cooked, remove and let cool. When cool enough to handle, carefully slice beets. If using canned beets, open can and drain out liquid. Place sliced beets, lentils, lemon juice, olive oil, basil, parsley, and salt in a bowl and toss well, coating all the beets. Divide arugula evenly between 6 plates. Place the beet and lentil mixture on top of the arugula. Sprinkle with crumbled goat cheese (if using) and serve.

CRISPY KALE

Kale is the new super-star vegetable. High in antioxidants, loaded with vitamin A and sulphur-containing, disease-fighting compounds, this nutritious vegetable has moved from the rear of the theater to center stage. Crispy Kale can be served as a side dish at lunch or dinner, or as a satisfying snack while at work or in the car.

SERVES: 2
EACH SERVING: 60 calories

INGREDIENTS:

1 large bunch of kale, washed and trimmed (3 cups)

Olive oil spray

1 T. kosher salt

2 T. pressed garlic

1 t. red pepper flakes

DIRECTIONS:

Preheat oven to 450°. Make sure kale is well washed and trimmed. Remove stems. Place on baking sheet. Spritz kale lightly with olive oil spray. Sprinkle with pressed garlic, kosher salt, and red pepper flakes. Bake in oven until crispy, approximately 12 minutes.

THE FAT-BLAST GROCERY LIST

You will be buying lots of produce, both fruits and vegetables, while on this diet (and for the rest of your life, I hope). This also means you will need a lot of refrigerator storage space. You might find yourself grocery shopping more often to accommodate the bulk of fresh produce.

Don't worry if you cannot purchase every item called for in each recipe. For instance, if you have broccoli on hand, but the recipe calls for cauliflower, substitute what you have in the fridge or freezer for the missing ingredient. Know that you can always substitute frozen for fresh if space, time, or money is a factor.

Because you might be mixing and matching days from different weeks, I thought it would be better to do a comprehensive overview of what is needed to follow the diet plan instead of a day-by-day or a week-by-week list. You can bring this book with you to the store and purchase the items for a few days at a time. This will allow you to use up leftovers and save money.

Also if there is a food you don't like, substitute something similar that you do like. If you have to leave out some of the ingredients due to cost or because they are not in the house, most of the recipes will still come out fine. My way of eating is just as much artistry as it is science!

It is important to know that you do not have to get each day's menu exactly right to see results. A few missing ingredients here and there will not dampen your weight loss. Flexibility is crucial for long-term weight maintenance, so learn to go with the flow during the 7-Day Fat-Blast Diet and don't let imperfection derail your long-term goals. This less-rigid approach increases your chance of weight-loss success. Most importantly, it is not whether you follow the diet to a T but rather that you don't stop the diet.

Skinny Pantry Staples

Nuts

Raw almonds
Pistachios
Raw walnuts
Raw pecans
Dry-roasted peanuts

Seeds

Raw pumpkin seeds
Raw sunflower seeds
Ground flaxseed
Chia seed

Sweets

Dark chocolate chips
Dark chocolate squares
Crystallized ginger
Maple syrup

Dried Fruits

Dried cherries
Dried cranberries
Dates

Jams

All natural fruit spreads

Oil and Vinegars

Red wine vinegar
Extra-virgin, cold-pressed olive
oil (store in refrigerator)
Toasted sesame oil

Beverages

Green tea
Coffee
Bottled water

Condiments

Mustard
Kosher salt
Red pepper flakes

Sauces

Tomato sauce
Salsa
Teriyaki sauce

Jarred Vegetables

Dill pickles
Roasted red peppers in a jar

Canned Goods

White albacore tuna
Lentils
Black beans
Kidney beans
Cannellini beans
Pineapple juice
Black olives
Artichoke hearts packed in water
Hearts of palm
Water chestnuts

Root Vegetables

Beets
Carrots
Parsnips
Jicama

Starchy Vegetables

Corn
Red potatoes
Sweet potatoes

Cruciferous Vegetables

Cabbage
Asian cabbage
Cauliflower
Kale
Broccoli

Green Leafy Vegetables

Spinach
Arugula
Romaine
Mixed greens
Iceberg lettuce
Kale

Other Vegetables

Mushrooms
Tomatoes
Red bell peppers
Cucumbers
Asparagus

Fennel bulb
Red onion
Eggplant
Celery
Zucchini
Pea pods
Spaghetti squash

Herbs, Onions, Garlic

Cilantro
Basil
White onions
Red onions
Shallots
Garlic

Fruits for Smoothies

Pineapple
Pineapple juice
Banana
Blueberries, strawberries,
raspberries
Frozen mango

Fruits for Snacks

Apples
Plums
Tangerines
Grapes
Pears
Dried cherries
Dried cranberries

Fruits for Salads

Mango
Avocado
Dried cranberries
Dried cherries

Fruit Juice

Orange juice
Pineapple juice

Proteins — Poultry

Chicken breasts
Turkey breasts
Turkey bacon
Ground turkey

Proteins — Shellfish

Shrimp
Scallops

Proteins — Fish

Salmon
Smoked Salmon
Tilapia

Proteins — Beef and Lamb

Lean ground beef
Flank steak
Loin of lamb

Proteins — Plant-based

Veggie burgers
Natural peanut butter

Lentils
Kidney beans
White beans
Black beans
Edamame
Tofu

Carbohydrates

Whole-wheat bread
Hummus
Whole-wheat spaghetti
Quinoa
Whole-wheat tortillas
Whole-grain hamburger buns
Corn tortillas
Baked tortilla chips
Baked potato chips
Whole-wheat bagels
Whole-grain crackers
Long-grain brown rice

Dairy

Low-fat cottage cheese
Low-fat yogurt
Part skim mozzarella
Low-fat cheddar cheese
Low-fat yogurt plain
Flavored low-fat yogurt
(90 calories)
Eggs or egg whites
Feta cheese
Parmesan
Non-fat skim milk
Goat cheese, semi soft
Low-fat cream cheese

SKINNY FOOD AND EXERCISE LOG

The only "perfect" fitness routine is the
one you can stick with!

—*Denise*

The Skinny Food and Exercise Log can help you be successful in blasting the fat and getting skinny and healthy! Studies have shown that keeping a written record of your progress (calories and amount of exercise) can actually help you lose weight and permanently keep off the pounds. It makes sense; keeping track of your calories in (food) and calories out (exercise) can help you be accountable for your weight-loss program.

Use the following spaces to record your daily food and beverage intake and your daily exercise intensity and time.

WEEK 1

DAY	FOOD/CALORIES	EXERCISES
Day 1		
Day 2		

WEEK 1

DAY	FOOD/CALORIES	EXERCISES
Day 3		
Day 4		

WEEK 1

DAY	FOOD/CALORIES	EXERCISES
Day 5		
Day 6		
Day 7		

WAIST MEASUREMENT: _____

WEEK 1 NOTES

FAVORITE FOODS

FAVORITE EXERCISES

WEEK 2

DAY	FOOD/CALORIES	EXERCISES
Day 1		
Day 2		

WEEK 2

DAY	FOOD/CALORIES	EXERCISES
Day 3		
Day 4		

WEEK 2

DAY	FOOD/CALORIES	EXERCISES
Day 5		
Day 6		
Day 7		

WAIST MEASUREMENT: _____

WEEK 2 NOTES

FAVORITE FOODS

FAVORITE EXERCISES

WEEK 3

DAY	FOOD/CALORIES	EXERCISES
Day 1		
Day 2		

WEEK 3

DAY	FOOD/CALORIES	EXERCISES
Day 3		
Day 4		

WEEK 3

DAY	FOOD/CALORIES	EXERCISES
Day 5		
Day 6		
Day 7		

WAIST MEASUREMENT: _____

WEEK 3 NOTES

FAVORITE FOODS

FAVORITE EXERCISES

WEEK 4

DAY	FOOD/CALORIES	EXERCISES
Day 1		
Day 2		

WEEK 4

DAY	FOOD/CALORIES	EXERCISES
Day 3		
Day 4		

WEEK 4

DAY	FOOD/CALORIES	EXERCISES
Day 5		
Day 6		
Day 7		

WAIST MEASUREMENT: _____

WEEK 4 NOTES

FAVORITE FOODS

FAVORITE EXERCISES

WEEK 5

DAY	FOOD/CALORIES	EXERCISES
Day 1		
Day 2		

WEEK 5

DAY	FOOD/CALORIES	EXERCISES
Day 3		
Day 4		

WEEK 5

DAY	FOOD/CALORIES	EXERCISES
Day 5		
Day 6		
Day 7		

WAIST MEASUREMENT: _____

WEEK 5 NOTES

FAVORITE FOODS

FAVORITE EXERCISES

WEEK 6

DAY	FOOD/CALORIES	EXERCISES
Day 1		
Day 2		

WEEK 6

DAY	FOOD/CALORIES	EXERCISES
Day 3		
Day 4		

WEEK 6

DAY	FOOD/CALORIES	EXERCISES
Day 5		
Day 6		
Day 7		

WAIST MEASUREMENT: _____

WEEK 6 NOTES

FAVORITE FOODS

FAVORITE EXERCISES

WEEK 7

DAY	FOOD/CALORIES	EXERCISES
Day 1		
Day 2		

WEEK 7

DAY	FOOD/CALORIES	EXERCISES
Day 3		
Day 4		

WEEK 7

DAY	FOOD/CALORIES	EXERCISES
Day 5		
Day 6		
Day 7		

WAIST MEASUREMENT: _____

WEEK 7 NOTES

FAVORITE FOODS

FAVORITE EXERCISES

WEEK 8

DAY	FOOD/CALORIES	EXERCISES
Day 1		
Day 2		

WEEK 8

DAY	FOOD/CALORIES	EXERCISES
Day 3		
Day 4		

WEEK 8

DAY	FOOD/CALORIES	EXERCISES
Day 5		
Day 6		
Day 7		

WAIST MEASUREMENT: _____

WEEK 8 NOTES

FAVORITE FOODS

FAVORITE EXERCISES

REFERENCES AND SUPPORTING RESOURCES

CHAPTER 1

Body mass index. Centers for Disease Control and Prevention Web site. *http://www.cdc.gov/healthyweight/assessing/bmi/.* September 13, 2012. Accessed October 11, 2012.

Golden, SH, Robinson, KA, Saldanha I, Anton B, Ladenson PW. Prevalence and incidence of endocrine and metabolic disorders in the United States: a Comprehensive Review. *J Clin Endocrinol Metab.* 2009 Jun;94(6):1853-78. Review.

Is your medicine cabinet making you fat? MedicineNet.com Web site. *http://www.medicinenet.com/script/main/art.asp?articlekey=56339.* November 2, 2005. Accessed October 11, 2012.

Physicians' Desk Reference. 64th ed. Montvale, NJ: PDR Network, 2010.

CHAPTER 3

Dietary supplement fact sheet: multivitamin/mineral supplements. Office of Dietary Supplements. National Institutes of Health. *http://ods.od.nih.gov/factsheets/MVMS-QuickFacts/.* Accessed October 11, 2012.

CHAPTER 4

Grøntved A, Rimm EB, Willett WC, Andersen LB, Hu FB. A prospective study of weight training and risk of type 2 diabetes mellitus in men. Arch Intern Med. 2012 Aug 6:1-7. doi: 10.1001/archinternmed.2012.3138. [Epub ahead of print].

Hatfield, Frederick C. Bodybuilding according to Joe Weider. *http://www.bodybuilding.com*. May 23, 2003. Accessed October 11, 2012.

CHAPTER 7

Dow CA, Going SB., Chow HH, Patil BS, Thomson CA. The effects of daily consumption of grapefruit on body weight, lipids, and blood pressure in healthy, overweight adults." *Metabolism.* 2012 Jul;61(7): 1026-35. Epub 2012 Feb 2.

Murray MT. *The Encyclopedia of Healing Foods. New York: Atria Books;* 2005.

Mansour MS, Ni YM, Roberts AL, Kelleman M, Roychoudhury A, St-Onge, MP. Ginger consumption enhances the thermic effect of food and promotes feelings of satiety without affecting metabolic and hormonal parameters in overweight men: a pilot study. *Metabolism.* 2012 Oct;61(10):1347-52.

Palmer, S. Understanding the Health Benefits of Tomato Products. SCANNERS. *http://www.tomatowellness.com/static/news/SCAN-SCANNERS-Fall09-Vol_2_No_2-Tomato_Products.pdf.* Fall 2009. Accessed October 11, 2012.

Calcium Content of Foods. UCSF Medical School. *http://www.ucsfhealth. org/education/calcium_content_of_selected_foods/index.html.* Accessed October 11, 2012.

CHAPTER 8

Alappat L, Awad, AB. Curcumin and obesity: evidence and mechanisms." *Nutr Rev.* 2010 Dec;68(12):729-38.

American Chemical Society (ACS). New evidence on effects of green coffee beans in weight loss. *http://www.sciencedaily.com/ releases/2012/03/120327134209.htm.* March 27, 2012. Retrieved October 11, 2012, from (2012, March 27).

American Physiological Society (2006, April 4). Pine nut oil boosts appetite suppressors up to 60 percent for 4 hours. *http://www*

.sciencedaily.com/releases/2006/04/060404085953.htm. April 4, 2006. Retrieved October 11, 2012.

Calorie count in pine nuts, pignolia, dried. *http://caloriecount.about.com/ calories-pine-nuts-pignolia-dried-i12147?size_grams=28.3*. Accessed October 11, 2012.

Weil, A. Naringenin: Drink more grapefruit juice? *http://www.drweil. com/drw/u/QAA400863/Naringenin-Drink-More-Grapefruit-Juice.html*. January 20, 2011. Accessed October 11, 2012.

Zółtaszek R, Hanausek M, Kiliańska ZM, Walaszek Z. [The biological role of D-glucaric acid and its derivatives: potential use in medicine]. [abstract] *Postepy Hig Med Dosw (Online)*. 2008 Sep 5;62:451-62. *http:// www.ncbi .nlm.nih.gov/pubmed?term=glucarates%2C%20breast*. Accessed October 11, 2012. PMID: 18772850.

Reinbach HC, Smeets A, Martinussen T, Moller P, and Westerterp-Plantenga MS. Effects of capsaicin, green tea, and CH-19 sweet pepper on appetite and energy intake in humans in negative and positive energy balance. *Clin Nutr*. 2009 Jun;28(3):260-5.

Nutrition Facts: Milk, fluid, nonfat, calcium fortified (fat free or skim). *http://nutritiondata.self.com/facts/dairy-and-egg-products/7578/2*. Accessed October 11, 2012.

Teegarden D, Zemel, MB. Dairy product components and weight regulation: symposium overview. *J Nutr*. 2003 Jan;133(1):243S-244S.

Guerreiro S, Monteiro R, Calhau C, Azevedo I, Soares R. Naringenin inhibits cell growth and migration in human breast cancer cell lines. [abstract] *FASEB*. 2007;21:848.5. *http://www.fasebj.org/cgi/content/ meeting_abstract/21/6/A1094-d*. Accessed October 11, 2012.

Tsi D, Nah AK, Kiso Y, Moritani T, Ono H. Clinical study on the combined effect of capsaicin, green tea extract and essence of chicken on body fat content in human subjects." *J Nutr Sci Vitaminol*. 2003 Dec;49(6):437–41.

Vinson JA, Burnham BR, and Nagendran MV. Randomized, double-blind, placebo-controlled, linear dose, crossover study to evaluate the efficacy and safety of a green coffee bean extract in overweight subjects." *Diabetes Metab Syndr Obes.* 2012;5:21-7.

CHAPTER 9

Levine, JA. Non-exercise activity thermogenesis (NEAT). *Best Pract Res Clin Endocrinol Metab.* 2002 Dec;16(4):679-702.

ABOUT THE AUTHOR

Denise Austin, often referred to as "America's favorite fitness expert," has sold over 25 million exercise videos and authored more than 10 books on health and fitness. As a worldwide fitness phenomenon, she has created a loyal audience with her top-rated fitness television shows: *Getting Fit*, which ran for 10 years on ESPN, and *Denise Austin's Daily Workout* and *Fit & Lite*, which both aired on Lifetime. Denise served two terms on the President's Council on Physical Fitness and Sports. She has testified before the U.S. Senate Committee on Health, Education, Labor and Pensions, helped launch the new food guidance system of the U.S. Department of Agriculture, and was recently honored by Woman's Day magazine and the American Heart Association with the Red Dress Award for her contributions to heart health. Married for over 25 years to Jeff Austin, they have two teenage daughters, Kelly and Katie.

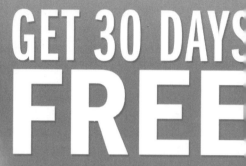